Fear in Cognitive Neuroscience

Fear in Cognitive Neuroscience

Salvatore Campanella
Editor

Nova Science Publishers, Inc.
New York

For permission to use material from this book please contact us:
Telephone 631-231-7269; Fax 631-231-8175
Web Site: http://www.novapublishers.com

Library of Congress Cataloging-in-Publication Data
Available upon request.

ISBN: 1-59454-502-2

Published by Nova Science Publishers, Inc. ✣New York

CONTENTS

In: Fear in Cognitive Neuroscience
Editor: Salvatore Campanella, pp. 1-6

ISBN: 1-59454-502-2

Chapter 1

WHAT COGNITIVE NEUROSCIENCES CAN TELL ABOUT THE EMOTION OF FEAR: A GENERAL INTRODUCTION

Salvatore Campanella
CHU Brugmann, Psychiatry Department, Brussels, Belgium

For over 60 years, ideas about emotion in neuroscience have been the matter of many debates. For instance, several studies have focused on a debate concerning whether the neural correlate of emotion involves separate neural processes for separate emotions, or an integrated neural network able to code all emotions (Calder et al., 2001). Recent studies have shown that specific brain injuries can cause selective impairments in the recognition of emotional facial expressions (e.g., Adolphs et al., 1994 ; Sprengelmeyer et al., 1996), and functional imaging research has revealed distinct neural correlates for emotion processing in healthy individuals (e.g., Morris et al., 1996 ; Hamann et al., 1999). As a matter of fact, patient-based research has shown that damage to the amygdala causes a disproportionate impairment in the recognition of fear, whereas abnormalities of the insula-basal ganglia regions affect the recognition of facial signals of disgust. This led several authors to consider that specific emotions are represented in distributed neural systems (e.g., Panksepp, 2003 ; Berridge, 2003), or, more precisely, that a limited number of emotions (generally including happiness, sadness, anger, fear and disgust) have a " basic " status and can be represented by specific neural activations. Another important debate concerns the status of emotion in cognition (Schulkin et al., 2003). At their birth (late 20th century), cognitive sciences intended to study human cognition by highlighting abstract rules that guided behavior by manipulating internal representations. As a consequence, mental representations and their structures defined the guiding framework of cognitive sciences, and emotions were considered as " secretory " (Rey, 1980), " bodily and less than rational " (Schulkin et al., 2003). However, several studies showed that emotional information processing can be competent, like other forms of reasoning, and can be fast and accurate (e.g., Baron, 1990 ; Gigerenzer, 1991). Nowadays, a large number of cognitive scientists have begun to accept the reality of emotions (e.g., Lane and Nadel, 1999), and suggested that emotional processes, at times, can be elegant forms of problem-solving (Schulkin et al., 2003), showing, furthermore, a relative overlap with the neural structures implied in cognitive processing (Davidson, 2003). Cognitive-emotional interactions are perfectly illustrated when human fear responses are considered (Armony et al., 1997). Indeed, neural representations of sensory events are susceptible to selective attentional modulation: the act of paying attention to one particular stimulus inhibits the neural representation of other stimuli (e.g., Maunsell, 1995). Therefore, a simultaneous threatening stimulus may fail to be processed if it occurs outside the focus of attention. The amygdala is thought to play a crucial role in emotional behavior (e.g., Morris et al., 1996 ; 1998), and it is suggested that this structure may, in this kind of situations, interrupt (via a direct thalamo-amygdala pathway) the attentional process and redirect attentional resources to the threatening stimulus (e.g., Ledoux, 1995). In other words, we are confronted with a " cognitive " information-processing system that should be able to set aside ongoing programs to take into account " emotional " signals representing a potential immediate danger. In other words, it can be argued that, currently, the cognitive revolution is gradually giving way to an emotion revolution (Panksepp, 2003). Indeed, the recent appearance of a major contribution to the emotion literature from the cognitively oriented tradition gives rise to a new area of research, entitled by Lane and Nadel (1999) " Cognitive Neuroscience of Emotion ", or more commonly, " Affective Neurosciences " (e.g., Davidson et al., 2002). Conducted from a neuroscience perspective, this new area intends to describe the normal functioning (and interactions) between emotional and cognitive processes, its main goal being to understand how the impairment of these processes could lead to different clinical conditions where pathology is associated with emotional disorders. Facial expressions are a mechanism through which internal emotional states and intentions become available as external signals. The inability to decode these signals has been related to important individual and interpersonal problems. Indeed, it has been shown, for instance, that many psychiatric illnesses, such as depression (e.g., Bouhuys, 2003), anxiety disorders (e.g., Mogg and Bradley, 2002), psychopathy (e.g., Ogloff and Wong, 1990), alcohol dependance (e.g., Philippot et al., 2003) and schizophrenia (e.g., Krings and Earnst, 2003), showed impaired recognition of facial emotional expressions. In other words, Affective Neurosciences touch the broad community of biobehavioral research, as it is relevant to all areas of psychology and to much of psychiatry: as a consequence, many authors consider now that it will be crucial in helping to understand normal and psychopathological phenomenons (Davidson, 2003).

Two major statements can be drawn from what precedes: (1) specific emotions are represented in distributed neural networks ; and (2) emotional and cognitive processes are subserved by (partly) overlapping neural circuits. The acceptance of the reality of emotions has generated a new intense debate concerning the functions of emotions. According to Seligman (1970), biological evolution has predisposed animals to learn more easily to form associations between some stimuli rather than others because such associations were instrumental in promoting survival. This view, influenced by Darwin (1872/1965), envisioned emotions in functional adaptive terms, so that emotions are seen as part of an information-processing system aiming to solve a problematic situation. According to this, the most compelling illustration, that had gathered the large body of evidence, is furnished by the processing of threatening signals and its related emotion, i.e. fear.

Fear is an emotion that is particularly important to human and animal existence. It is a reaction to threatening events and is elicited when self-preservation goals are posed in danger during the pursuit of actions directed at other goals. A common view of fear in the neuroscience literature is that fear triggers the "fight or flight" response, characterized by increased heart rate, breathing, and muscle tension, which allows the individual to escape from danger or defend itself against a predator or conspecific (LeDoux, 1995; Ohman and Mineka, 2001). Based on the presence or absence of a stimulus, the brain regulates the strength and duration of this apparent coping mechanism. When this regulatory system malfunctions, however, it can lead to excessive fearfulness in certain individuals. Excessively fearful individuals appear to have difficulty suppressing the body's response to stress.

Fear is a complex phenomenon, and its complexity is manifested first and foremost in its being multi-component and multi-leveled. This will be exemplified in the following chapters, which will try to give us insights from the different neuroscientific perspectives from which fear is studied. This will also exemplify how the convergence between research at the animal level on the neural substrates of basic emotional processes and at the human level using neuroimaging and lesion methods has helped to establish a solid foundation upon which were built the " Affective Neurosciences " (Davidson, 2003).

The basis of emotional processing has been studied extensively in experimental animals by using a procedure pioneered by Pavlov, i.e. fear conditioning. The scope of these studies was to elicit fear responses after a meaningless stimulus (such as a light or a tone) occurs in connection with an aversive event (generally a mild shock). One of the main goals in cognitive neurosciences is to explain the relation between neural activity and behavior. With this in mind, a great part of these studies have focused on the role of the amygdala in fearful processing, showing that lesions of this structure interfere with the acquisition and the expression of various indices of conditioned fear. However, if many evidence were gathered thanks to animal research to assess the principal role of amygdala in fear processing, showing that the amygdala plays a similar role in humans has been difficult (Helmuth, 2003). In *Chapter 2*, Damien Debatisse and his colleagues (from the NeuroSurgical and Neurophysiological Unit of the Universitary Hospital of Lausanne, Switzerland) will give us an overview of the general findings as concerns the neural pathways devoted in animals in fear processing and pain avoidance in order to conclude with a global representation of the neurophysiological mechanisms implied in humans to process fear signals.

When the concept of fear is envisaged in neurosciences, it is necessarily referred to the amygdala, this almond-shape structure which is located deep within the brain. The second chapter will give us some insights about how this structure governs the abilities to experience fear and avoid pain through distributed neural circuits by focusing on a description of basic neurophysiological mechanisms. However, Cognitive Neurosciences can also furnish others levels of analysis. Indeed, Cognitive Psychology is interested since its birth by abstract rules governing mental representations in order to guide behaviors, and Cognitive Neurosciences try to link these mental processes to specific neural correlates by using brain imagery techniques. In *Chapter 3*, Céline Douilliez and Pierre Philippot (from the Emotion and Cognition Unit of the University of Louvain, Belgium) will specify the classical cognitive steps involved in emotional processing in order then to define the specific " cognitive " deficits involved in the process of fear signals in a psychopathological state such as anxiety. In *Chapter 4*, Gilles Pourtois and Patrick Vuillemier (from the Cognitive Neurosciences Department, University of Geneva, Switzerland) will focus on brain imagery results, in an attempt to show how the amygdala appears to intercede between emotion and attention in two related ways. The first one suggests that signals from the amygdala enhance the processing of fear-inducing images by higher level cortical regions. The second one is more controversial and suggests that the amgygdala can also operate without communication from higher visual areas.

Most of the current works investigating the neural basis of emotions try to identify the neural structures for the experience or expression of particular emotions. Rather, emotions can also be characterized by patterns of neuromodulations of certain sets of brain structures included in broad neural network. Indeed, for instance, it has been shown that conditioned effects often depend on N-methyl-D-aspartate receptor activation within the basolateral amygdala when initially neutral stimuli are paired with emotionally significant stimuli, such as shocks or food (Davis and Whalen, 2001). In *Chapter 5*, Emmanuel Streel and his colleagues (from the Addiction Unit of the University of Brussels, Belgium) will show us how the emotion of fear could also be conceptualized at a more molecular level.

Finally, as suggested above, many psychiatric diseases present specific deficits in the decoding of emotions. In *Chapter 6*, Alfredo Velardi and his colleagues will show us how deficits in the decoding of the fear emotion could be linked with some particular form of mood disorders, such as different forms of anxiety. In *Chapter 7*, Laurent Servais and his collaborators will give us some insights about the relations that have been described between a deficit in the decoding of fear emotion and some psychopathological states, such as antisocial personnalities and/or psychopathy.

Overall, these chapters will try to give us a general overview of how the fear emotion is nowadays conceptualized in the growing area of Cognitive Neurosciences. To do so, animal and human studies including experimental, pharmacological, neurophysiological and brain imagery experiments will be reported, with the principal aim to show (1) the neurophysiological (Chapter 2) and neuroanatomical (Chapter 4) structures implied in the decoding of the fear emotion ; (2) their relationships with the different cognitive steps implied in this function (Chapter 3) and their pharmacological functioning (Chapter 5) ; and (3) the relations existing between a deficit in the decoding of this fear emotion and some pathological states such as anxiety (Chapters 2,3 and 6) and psychopathy (Chapter 7). We are aware that this contribution would be minimal, as many other domains and data could have been reported. However, this book is an interesting attempt to put together different data coming from different areas of Cognitive Neurosciences, and we are convinced that important contributions in the understanding of human cognition can only be realized through multidisciplinary collaborations.

REFERENCES

Adolphs, R., Tranel, D., Damasio, H., and Damasio, A.R. (1994). Impaired recognition of emotional facial expressions following bilateral damage to the human amygdala. *Nature,* 372, 669-672.

Armony, J.L., Servan-Schreiber, D., Cohen, J.D., and Ledoux, J.E. (1997). Computational modeling of emotion: explorations through the anatomy and physiology of fear conditioning. *Trends in Cognitive Sciences,* 1, 28-34.

Baron, J. (1990). Thinking and deciding. Cambridge: Cambridge University Press.

Berridge, K.C. (2003). Pleasures of the brain. *Brain and Cognition,* 52, 106-128.

Bouhuys, A.L. (2003). Ethology and depression. In Philippot, P., Feldman, R.S., and Coats, E.J. (Eds.), *Nonverbal behavior in clinical settings.* New York: Oxford University Press.

Calder, A.J., Lawrence, A.D., and Young, A.W. (2001). Neuropsychology of fear and loathing. *Nature Reviews,* 2, 352-363.

Darwin, C. (1872/1965). The expression of emotions. Chicago: University of Chicago Press.

Davidson, R.J., Pizzagalli, D., Nitschke, J.B., and Putnam, K.M. (2002). Depression: Perspectives from affective neurosciences. *Annual review of Psychology*, 53, 545-574.

Davidson, R.J. (2003). Seven sins in the study of emotion: Correctives from affective neuroscience. *Brain and Cognition,* 52, 129-132.

Davis, M., and Whalen, P.J. (2001). The amygdala: vigilance and emotion. *Molecular Psychiatry,* 6, 13-34.

Gigerenzer, G. (1991). From tools to theories: A heuristic of discovery in cognitive psychology. *Psychological Review,* 98, 254-267.

Hamann, S.B., Ely, T.D., Grafton, S.T., and Kilts, C.D. (1999). Amygdala activity related to enhanced memory for pleasant and aversive memory. *Nature Neuroscience,* 2, 289-293.

Helmuth, L. (2003). Cognitive neuroscience. Fear and trembling in the amygdala. *Science,* 300, 568-569.

Kring, A.M., and Earnst, K.S. (2003). Nonverbal behavior in schizophrenia. In Philippot, P., Feldman, R.S., and Coats, E.J. (Eds.), *Nonverbal behavior in clinical settings.* New York: Oxford University Press.

Lane, R.D., and Nadel, L. (Eds.). (1999). *Cognitive neuroscience of emotion.* New York, NY: Oxford University Press.

Ledoux, J.E. (1995). Emotions: clues from the brain. *Annual Review of Psychology,* 46, 209-235.

Maunsell, J.H.R. (1995). The brain's visual world: representation of visual targets in cerebral cortex. *Science,* 270, 764-769.

Mogg, K., and Bradley, B.P. (2003). Selective processing of nonverbal information in anxiety: attentional biases for threat. In Philippot, P., Feldman, R.S., and Coats, E.J. (Eds.), *Nonverbal behavior in clinical settings.* New York: Oxford University Press.

Morris, J.S., Frith, C.D., Perrett, D.I., Rowland, D., Young, A.W., Calder, A.J., and Dolan, R.J. (1996). A differential neural response in the human amygdala to fearful and happy facial expressions. *Nature,* 383, 812-815.

Morris, J.S., Ohman, A., and Dolan, R.J. (1998). Conscious and unconscious emotional learning in the human amygdala. *Nature,* 393, 467-470.

Ogloff, J.R., and Wong, S. (1990). Electrodermal and cardiovascular evidence of a coping response in psychopaths. *Criminal Justice and Behaviour*, 17, 231-245.

Ohman, A., and Mineka, S. (2001). Fears, phobias, and preparedness: toward an evolved module of fear and fear learning. *Psychological Review,* 108(3), 483-522.

Panksepp, J. (2003). At the interface of the affective, behavioral, a,d cognitive neurosciences: Decoding the emotional feelings of the brain. *Brain and Cognition*, 52, 4-14.

Philippot, P., Kornreich, C., and Blairy, S. (2003). Nonverbal deficits and interpersonal regulation in alcoholics. In Philippot, P., Feldman, R.S., and Coats, E.J. (Eds.), *Nonverbal behavior in clinical settings.* New York: Oxford University Press.

Rey, G. (1980). Functionalism and the emotions. In E.O. Rorty (Ed.), Explaining *the emotions* (pp. 163-196). Berkeley, CA: University of California Press.

Schulkin, J., Thompson, B.L., and Rosen, J.B. (2003). Demythologizing the emotions: Adaptation, cognition, and visceral representations of emotion in the nervous system. *Brain and Cognition,* 52, 15-23.

Seligman, M.E.P. (1970). On the generality of laws of learning. *Psychological Review,* 77, 406-418.

Sprengelmeyer R, Young AW, Calder AJ, Karnat A, Lange H, Homberg V, Perrett DI, Rowland D. (1996). Loss of disgust. Perception of faces and emotions in Huntington's disease. *Brain,* 119, 1647-65.

In: Fear in Cognitive Neuroscience
Editor: Salvatore Campanella, pp. 7-34
ISBN: 1-59454-502-2

Chapter 2

EMOTIONS, FEAR AND FRIGHT IN THE HUMAN BEING

D. Debatisse[1], E. Pralong[1], S. Bolyn[2], P. A. Despland[2], J. Ghika[2] and J. G. Villemure[1]
[1] UNN Neurosurgery and the Neurology Department
[2] CHUV Lausanne, Switzerland

FOREWORD

"Tale" of fear and fright, this one taken from "real-life experience":

> An excerpt from "Don't be scared of knowing - Rwanda: one million dead". In this book published by Robert Laffont, Yolande Mukagasama, a Tutsi girl who survived the genocide reports: " ...Very quietly then, one of them slapped my face and ordered: "Open your mouth!" I opened my mouth. "Wider!" I made an effort. "Wider!" and suddenly he unfastened a grenade from his belt and he pushed it into my mouth. My mouth was too small. He punched me and the grenade sank in, breaking my teeth. I suddenly went mad. I started running all over the place among the laughing soldiers. I kept on trying to remove the grenade, but I just couldn't do it. It was stuck in my mouth like some too big fruit. I was running like hell, a stream of memories was passing through my mind; back to my mind too, children falling into their graves... "

This extract of course urges us to think about every single brain structure level enabling us to get a better understanding of the mechanisms of fear and fright but also forces us to answer the following question: has man changed since the dawn of mankind ? In other words: with our supposedly evolved brain, are we still identical human beings as far as our behaviours and emotions are concerned? Are we going to evolve towards "different" behaviours? One point is sure: some emotions make us "develop", other ones lead us to doubt about the difference between man and animal.

1. Introduction

Fear and fright are definitely products of the emotional concept and are part and parcel of the province of emotions. As these emotions (fear and fright) are relatively little known, we will start with a short historical, neuro-anatomic and "biological" reminder in order to reach a better understanding of the afferent and involved brain structures. A thorough knowledge of these two emotions might enable us to determine the origin of these outward signs. Over the past two decades, there was a rapid development of new techniques in the fields of functional imaging, neurophysiology and neurosciences in general. There is thus no limit now to what we can hope for at the dawn of the third millennium. We can come to enhanced modelling (too reductionist up to now). We can above all– with all humility - fairly master multiple neural networks (of the human being as a whole too) accounting for what we are now: men and living creatures (mammals), able to think in an abstract way and fairly ass°Ling their frights and anxieties. Better knowledge of this should help us to participate in Man such as we will be tomorrow.

1.1. A Little Bit of History

There is nothing new at all in locating mental functions within the brain. More than 200 years ago, Franz Joseph Gall (1758-1728) established the fundaments of phrenology. He believed that intellectual and moral faculties were innate and that their manifestation depended on the organisation of the brain. Every feeling or mental faculty was supposed to be dependent of a more or less developed brain "organ", an internal development with repercussions on the shape of the skull (in French, they say "avoir la bosse des maths" - literally: to have a bum for maths – to speak of a person who has a gift for maths).

In the early 19th century, Walter Cannon (1871-1945), especially famous for his attacks against William James's emotion theory, also made a few joint experiments with Philip Bard with a view to find a brain substratum to emotions. They found a series of strategic lesions, which brought them to the conclusion that the hypothalamus was the central part of the "emotion brain". Recognising this status of centre of emotions was quite logical given its position between the evolutionarily refined cortex and the primitive sub-cortical structures; furthermore they already knew about the part it played in the regulation of the autonomous nervous system. Then, in 1937, James Papez (1883-1958), an anatomist, set forth one of the most influential theories on the brain substratum of emotions. Papez was influenced by the work of C. Judson Herrick, a specialist of evolution, who had made a distinction between the side parts and the medium parts of the cortex. According to him, the medium cortex was originally much older than the side cortex. Papez, who had a comprehensive approach, merged the ideas of Herrick and the research work on hypothalamus and on internal injuries. He thus came to a theory that explained the subjective feeling of emotions by a flow of information through a circuit interconnecting the hypothalamus to the median cortex. This circuit is still known today as *Papez's circuit*. Unlike Cannon, who considered the hypothalamus to be a homogeneous structure, Papez distinguished a sub-region called mammillary body (because it protrudes like breasts). He thought that region was the only one that received the sensory message from the thalamus and passed it on to the cingular cortex through the anterior nucleus of the thalamus. He also clearly pointed to the hippocampus as the receiver of outputs from the cingular cortex, which thus closed the loop by sending messages to the mammillary body through the fornix. Papez suggested that emotions could be generated by two ways through this circuit: on the one hand by sensory stimuli entering through the thalamus and successively crossing the various structures of the circuit we have just described; on the other hand by thoughts coming from the cortex, which integrate into the circuit through the cingular cortex. Papez's circuit was a brilliant attempt to explain emotions by the anatomic tracts. Although very few techniques were available at the time to study the brain track, virtually all the tracts forecast by Papez turned out to be real. Unfortunately for him, very few of these tracts are recognised today as being involved in emotions; they are rather involved in circuits concerning the declarative memory. This being said, there is no doubt about the historic importance of Papez's circuit as it was to be at the origin of the limbic system theory. Research work on the brain bases of emotions was slowed down by World War II, but it knew an important advance in 1949, when Paul MacLean revisited Papez's circuit and made it more complex. He believed that the rhinencephalon – i.e. this old part of the cortex involved in olfaction - played a central role in emotions, especially as it made important connections with the hypothalamus. It remained relatively important in the human being where olfaction is a rather atrophied sense compared to other species. As he had noticed that stimulating the rhinencephalon produced visceral responses similar to those provoked by emotions, MacLean decided to turn it into its emotion "centre". He paid a particular importance to the hippocampus, comparing its well-aligned pyramidal neurones to an "emotional keyboard" receiving its messages both from the outside world and from the inner world. MacLean believed that integrating these two types of sensations was at the basis of emotional experience. In 1952, MacLean introduced the term "limbic system" to designate the visceral brain of the rhinencephalon . The word "limbic" had been introduced by Paul Pierre Broca (1824-1880), a French anatomist, to designate the median part of the cortex which has the shape of a ring (from Latin limbus, brim). MacLean believed that the limbic system included not only Papez's circuit, but also regions like the amygdala, the septum and the forefront cortex. All these structures were supposed to form a phylogenetically old integrated system assuring the survival of the individual thanks to adapted visceral and affective responses. In 1970, MacLean introduced his "triunic brain" theory, according to which the brain passed through three evolution stages: reptilian, paleomammalian and neomammalian. The three brains are present together in the human being and in the more evolved mammals. The most primitive vertebrates only have a paleomammalian and a reptilian brain whereas birds, reptiles, amphibians and fishes just have a reptilian brain. The neomammalian brain – corresponding essentially to the limbic system – is to be found in all mammals. Since then, especially over the last two decades, neurology and neuroscience have progressed in the knowledge of the anatomic substrata involving mental functions and emotions. It is thus now possible to trace back the "channels" leading to them, resulting in a more efficient, sophisticated and scientific understanding of these phenomena. Through animal experiments followed by the application of theoretical models on human beings, neurosciences took up studying brain pathologies in clinical situations (often caused by a lesion). More recently, techniques based on functional imaging and neurophysiological exploration enabled us to visualise how the brain works in a given situation (for example, motor and cognitive tasks, mental states or emotions...). Speaking of emotions, the problem is: how can we define an emotion?

1.2. What is an Emotion?

Defining what is an emotion is by no means an easy task, as we have to characterise with words manifestations that are linked with a mental experience, which is of course essentially subject to physical manifestations felt at body level. While the concept of emotion is an object of popular and universal knowledge, it remains quite approximately defined, as it mainly opens up to a vast and poorly delimited semantic field. From an etymological point of view, the word emotion comes from Latin *ex movere*, which means an outward movement, but this definition will not help us. Nevertheless, this first approach suggests that the fact to incite to action can bring about intense affective conditions that will then be called emotions. According to numerous clinical and neurobiological data, it would seem that the so-called "emotional" processes would play an essential part in the psychic dynamics of the human being for the following reasons: Emotions are structural, they are inextricably linked to the functional dynamics of the central nervous system. They play an important and essential role: they interfere in elaborating the affective state and behaviours, they alter or disturb cognitive faculties and influence our health condition. Suppressing or altering them is impossible (it is only possible to modulate existing emotions). Most often, emotions are very difficult to control, as emotional processes are automatic, involuntary, quickly variable and "infectious". Numerous factors lead to emotions: *Internal factors:* cognitive and physiological processes, deficiency of psychic needs (~ affective needs), pathology or trauma of the CNS. *External factors:* aggression, various accidental factors.

1.3. Emotions Occur Steadily – In All Social Groups, in All People and in All Circumstances

At the individual level, an intensely emotional real-life experience is supposed to be perturbing: relationship towards oneself, relationships towards the outside world (and so, subsequently, socialisation). *At social level, an intensely emotional real-life experience is supposed to be perturbing:* through an "infection" phenomenon of the emotional state of the people in the group; group dynamics (and so, subsequently, the affective state of each person and the collective activities).

1.4. Emotion in the Dictionary

The word "emotion" is defined as an intense emotional state characterised by a sudden physical and mental disruption where, in the presence of some very sharp stimulation or representations, the appropriate reactions of adapting to the environment stop working. The *Shorter Oxford Dictionary* also gives the following definitions: a physical agitation or disturbance; agitation of mind; strong mental feeling; any of the natural instinctive affections of the mind (e.g. love, horror, pity) which come and go according to one's personality, experience and physical state; a mental feeling. Also, mental feeling as distinguished from knowledge and from will.

Fear: Fear is an unpleasant feeling of perceived risk or danger, real or not. Fear also can be described as a feeling of extreme dislike to some conditions/objects, such as: fear of darkness, fear of ghosts, etc. It is one of the basic emotions.

Fright: sudden fear, violent terror; alarm; anything (real or imaginary) that inspires terror; a person or thing of a grotesque or ridiculous appearance. *You gave me a dreadful fright!*

Synonyms:

agony, alarm, alert, anguish, anxiety, apprehension, commotion, confusion, dismay, fear, horror, jitters, panic, scare, shaking, terror, throes, trance, trembling.

1.5. Damasio's Model (1994)

Damasio's model (1994) defines emotions as configurations of chemical and neural responses whose aim is to help the body to keep alive by inducing adaptive behaviours. We can trace back all these phenomena over the phylogenesis whose result is man as we are now. So, these are the results of activating a set of cerebral structures, most of which are also involved in controlling and regulating bodily states around optimal physiological values. This is referred to as homeostasis.

"Damasio suggests that visually recognising facial expressions of emotion will engage regions in the right hemisphere that subserve both (1) visual representations of the perceptual properties of facial expressions ; (2) somatosensory representations of the emotion associated with such expressions ; and (3) additional regions (and white matter) that serve to link these two components. This composite visuosomatic system could permit attribution of mental states to other individuals, in part, by simulation of their visually observed body state. This interpretation is consonant with the finding that producing facial expressions by volitional contraction of specific muscles induces components of the emotional state normally associated with that expression (Adelmann and Zajonc, 1989; Levenson et al., 1990). It is also consonant with the finding of spontaneous facial mimicry in infants (Meltzoff and Moore, 1983). However, it is important to note that the comprehensive evocation of emotional feelings could be achieved without the need for actual facial mimicry, by the central generation of a somatosensory image, a process we have termed the "as-if loop" (Damasio, 1994). The finding of a disproportionately critical role for the right somatosensory-related cortices identifying emotions may also be related to the observation that damage to those regions can result in anosognosia, an impaired knowledge of one's own body state, often accompanied by a flattening of emotion (Babinski, 1914; Damasio, 1994). It remains unclear precisely which components of the somatosensory cortex would be most important in our task: those regions that represent the face or additional regions that could provide more comprehensive knowledge about the state of the entire body associated with an emotion."

2. Emotions, Fear, Fright and Biology

Emotions, but also fear and the sensation of fright, are biologically determined, stereotyped and automatic, whereas the patient's individual culture, as well as his development are likely to influence all emotional inductors and to change the overt expression of emotions and fright.

2.1. Categorising Emotions

Ekman (1990) distinguishes 6 types of primary or universal emotions, which can be perceived on facial expressions: joy, sadness, fear, anger, surprise and disgust. Other types of secondary and social emotions, such as jealousy, guilt or pride, will then be classified as background emotions: well-being or ill-being, quiet or tension, fatigue or energy. Inducing this type of emotion class is generally an internal affair. *There is therefore no univocal definition of the emotion concept.* We will then keep to the fact that a multicomponent brain process can be triggered by internal or external afferences and that it comes into expression on various axes. At this stage, we will also cling to the concept that fear and fright, considered as an internal and subjective feeling, correspond to a brain experience: an individual can experience quite a series of emotions, among which fright. Nevertheless, emotion is also a state of physiological awakening. Like all emotions, fear and fright are accompanied by a range of visceral and autonomous body reactions (such as modified heart rate, feeling of oesophageal constriction...). According to the type of emotion, *various behaviours* will be emphasised resulting, among other things, in *defence or attack* behaviours, or motor expressions of body movement mimicry, prosody, vocalisation or other symptoms. Last but not least: we will define an emotion as being short-lived and characterised by a sudden and momentary interruption of the affective balance. Should the situation persist, we will no longer speak of emotion, but of feeling.

2.2. Fear and Fright: "Pejorative" Terms Belonging to the Range of Emotions

Since the beginning of time, passions and emotions have been assimilated to the sway of the body over the spirit and their unsettling for instance is at the origin of madness. The traditional European point of view, which started with Empedocles (5th century BC), continued with Hippocrates and Galen and lasted up to the 17th century, was that our constitution depended on the balance of four humours – blood, yellow gall, black gall and pituita, which were supposed to circulate in the cavity of our body. Until recently, this kind of definition led us to consider four categories and four basic characters: sanguine, quick-tempered, melancholic and phlegmatic. Not until the 19th century did this point of view change, when it was considered that emotions were sublimated in the brain but kept their fluid species, an urge repressed in the unconscious depths of memory and likely to emerge as a source of anxiety and guilt, thus causing us to submit our will to their influence. In spite of the development of neuroscience, it is still difficult today to admit that an emotion could be a full-part brain function, moreover useful to the development of the brain and to its future as part of its timeless evolution. So the word emotion is generally regarded as pejorative and is often defined in dictionaries as *a disorder*. Basically, we will keep in mind that emotions – e.g. fear and more specifically fright – evoke a momentary loss of voluntary control of perception and behaviour.

2.3. Emotions, Fear and Fright from a Clinical Point of View

In human clinic – whatever the specialisation may be – the word "emotions" also designates temper diseases, anxiety, depressions leading to impulsive acts or to a behaviour quite unsuited to a situation. An intense emotion (e.g. fright) can disrupt the way of thinking and of acting of an individual and result in stereotyped or uncoordinated sequences; on the psychiatric and psychoanalytic side, an emotion can also divert its course and cause slips of the tongue or abortive actions. Nevertheless, emotions remain the representation of the emergence of drives or instincts of an "animal" type and are to be found in every population of more or less "developed" mammals – including man (see chapter: psychology)

2.4. Emotions, Fear and Fright – Vital Functions that are Necessary and Useful to the Brain

Emotions (the commonest ones being fear and fright, joy and sadness) are a major function of the brain, enabling this "central organ" to be informed on the internal state of the body, i.e. its vital needs, and on the values of external stimuli in terms of life and survival. Emotions also give an individual the possibility of letting other people know about the state of his internal assessment by using another channel than language or any other way of communication. In his book *"The expression of emotion in animals"*, published in 1865, Darwin (1809-1882) already emphasised that biological urges, like sex drives, aggressiveness or fear were good examples of emotional behaviour philo-genetically shared among the various animal species – including man. He considered this type of emotions to be essential to the preservation of the individual and of the species. The regulation of these so-called "archaic" drives is supposed to have been privileged by natural selection and has probably been the driving force behind the evolution of our brain, the one I am using to write these lines. So, there would have been no point developing a brain with a high memory or calculation capacity without a stimulation to act and react wisely according to the right time to guarantee its survival. It is therefore the ability of the central nervous system to create stimuli that has been the evolution priority for the 21st century brain. Emotions, fear and fright are initiated by one or several stimuli (real or imaginary) and lead to a perception involving processes such as identification, memory and specific associations. This emotional perception thus initiates a psychic experience which is not always conscious or likely to be verbalised, but which participates uppermost in impulsive or calculated decision-making. So, emotions, fear and fright make it possible to organise priorities into a hierarchy and get together to achieve an aim compatible with the notion of survival. These emotions can then lead to an intense motivation state and maintain it long enough to influence behaviour towards satisfying some internal need or acquiring some social advantage.

2.5. Emotions, Fear, Fright and Neurosciences – The "Lesion" Model

For a few decades neuropsychology and neurosciences have enabled us to understand, through the "lesion" model, how emotions – i.a. fear and fright – work. The most significant historic contributions include:

- **Sham Rage**-One of the first experimental demonstrations of the relationships between brain and emotions was achieved in the early 20th century by Cannon and Bart, who established that surgical ablation of a cat's neocortex led to an aggressive and non-motivated behaviour (Sham Rage). These decerebrated animals react to trivial stimuli by grunting growling and intense gut reactions showing that their emotional reactivity is no longer inhibited by the cortex.
- **Klüver-Bucy's syndrome**-As early as 1938, research work carried out by Klüver and Lean brought about a significant advance in understanding the links between brain and emotions. They gave the first experimental evidence of the implication of a part of the brain in regulating the emotional behaviour while performing on apes bilateral ablation of vast portions of the temporal lobe including the amygdala, the hippocampus and an important part of the neocortex in apes. Those lobectomised animals behaved in a docile and submissive way, they experienced fearing loss, hypersexuality, general hyperorality and reactions of enhanced vigilance to any visual stimulus despite visual identification disorders such as visual agnosia. This kind of syndrome can appear following various diseases affecting temporal lobes (herpetic encephalitis or certain degenerative diseases).
- **Phineas Gage (1823-1860)**-The case of this patient is also well documented and rather famous in the literature of emotions. In 1848, in New England, this twenty-five-year old man was a victim of an accident at work: an iron bar entered his left jaw, crossed the basis of his skull and the front of his brain and finally went out at the top of his head, causing lesions to the ventral and median regions of his frontal lobes. During the regression phase of this accident, his personality underwent radical changes while his cognitive functions remained unchanged. He used to be a serious young man, famous for his conscientiousness, his moderation and his strength of character. Following that accident, he became rude, whimsical, and impulsive and he always had moods. We can learn a lot from this first case, especially about the links between personality and the past of the frontal lobe. It shows that even if his intellectual abilities are intact, an individual can become unable to use his judgement faculties in everyday life and to adapt his behaviour to choices. Following this accident, Gage eventually developed incompetence in social relationships and was no longer able to make consistent and targeted decisions.
- **Urbach-Wiethe's syndrome**-Identifying emotions: spontaneous bilateral destruction of amygdalas causes the disease of Urbach-Wiethe, characterised by the inability to identify emotions after facial expressions. As we know, the various expressions of the face reflect emotions that can be easily identified. Amygdalas therefore play a role in deciphering the feelings of another person (including in a love relationship!). Stimulating the amygdala brings about learning motivated by fear. The amygdala gives stimuli a character of aversion and triggers conditioning to fear.

3. Anatomic Reminder of the Nervous Structures Occurring in Emotions (Including Fear and Fright) in the Human Being

We should first of all recall that all structures that are going to be described are of course interconnected and that none of them is responsible for a specific emotional state and more specially for fear and fright. This interconnectivity and this simultaneous and multidirectional implication will prevent us from formally determining a simple, reductionist or linear representation of emotional processes, which makes very difficult a comprehensive conceptualisation of sequences and of the levels of information processing.

3.1. Papez's Circuit

In 1937, James Papez suggested and described a neural circuit to which he gave his name. It was supposed to be the minimum required anatomic substrate for emotions, among which fear and fright. His theory was essentially based on the post-mortem examination of brains of people suffering from affective disorders. He closely analysed the damaged structures he thought to be at the origin of their altered emotional behaviour. He then deduced that emotional experience depended on hippocampo-mamillo-thalamo-cingular circuits which later proved out to be essentially involved in the mnesic functions. Paul MacLean eventually took up Papez's ideas, this time associating the concept of the limbic lobe created by Broca. This concept suggests the notion of limbic system to which he attributes most affective functions and this in an evolutionist perspective. He considered that the human brain could be the evolutionary result of three systems having a concentric anatomic localisation:

1. **The reptilian brain** consists of the brainstem and the central grey nuclei that make up the oldest and deepest layer. This system controls the highly stereotyped actions enabling the individual to survive (eating, breathing, ...).
2. **The paleo-mammalian brain** corresponds to the limbic system. This second layer, which shrouds the reptilian nucleus, is supposed to play the role of preserving the species as well as the individual. This system consists of three subdivisions: an amygdalian one associated with self-preservation, a septal one linked to procreation and preservation of the species and a thalamo-cingular one involved in certain social and family relationships.
3. **The neo-mammalian brain** is the third and last layer and is only to be found in the so-called "superior" animals. This system consists of the neocortex and is supposed to be the seat of rational thinking; it should to some extent enable the individual not to be dependent on emotions anymore. Later a series of various brain regions were regrouped under the term of *limbic structures*. The point of convergence of all these different structures lies in their simplified microscopic architecture, the allocortex, as opposed to the rest of the cortex, the isocortex. The influence of the various limbic structures exerted on the hippocampus and on the temporal lobe occurs through Papez's circuit, also referred to as the hippocampo-mamillo-thalamic circuit. This refers to a subset of numerous connections linking limbic structures between

themselves. Fig. 2 shows how the information passes through them from the hippocampus to the mammillary bodies of the hypothalamus, then to the front nucleus of the thalamus, to the cingular cortex, then to the entorhinal cortex to finally come back to the hippocampus After being finally "passed on" several times in Papez's circuit, temporary associations, consisting of a set of cortical neurones generated by a particular event, are going to undergo some physical remodelling aimed at consolidating them. After some time (probably a few hours) these associations will then become stabilised and independent of the hippocampus. Bilateral lesion of the hippocampus will stop the formation of new long-term memories but will not erase those that had been encoded before the accident. With this gradual withdrawal of the limbic system, memories no longer pass through Papez's circuit; they are encoded in specific areas of the cortex corresponding to the areas where the sensory information at the origin of memories has been stored (the occipital cortex for visual memories, the temporal cortex for auditory ones, etc.). Mnesic traces passing through the cortex can last for decades, even for life.

3.2. What the Current Limbic System Includes:

Limbic structures properly speaking, i.e. the piriform lobe, include the hippocampus formation, the basal forebrain (nucleus basalis of Meynert, the nucleus of the septum), the ventral striatum and the amygdala.

Paralimbic structures make up the cortical part of the system and include the parahippocampus gyrus, the cingular gyrus, the retrospenial cortex, the septal area and finally structures that are considered to be related to the limbic system in view of their connection with some previously described areas, including the ventral tegmental of the mesencephalon, some thalamic nuclei (median and front ventral nuclei) and the hypothalamus.

3.3. Definitions of These Various Structures and Their Localisation

3.3.1. The Hypothalamus

The hypothalamus is a set of grey matter nuclei located next to the median face on the diencephalon on either side of the third ventricle. This latter has a lot of connections with the other prosencephalic structures and with the mesencephalon. The hypothalamus is the starting-point of the vegetative manifestations (quickening or slowing down of the heart rate, respiratory, digestive, sudoral, vasomotor changes) accompanying emotional reactions. The hypothalamus secretes several hormones, among which the releasing hormones, so called because they are likely to control the release of hormones by the pituitary gland and more particularly by its front part, the antehypophysis. Releasing hormones are secreted in a system of capillaries situated in the pituitary stem, which links the pituitary gland to the hypothalamus.

The hypothalamus has a major function in the vegetative life of the body as it acts on how viscera operate by interfering i.a. on the respiratory track and the heart system. It also controls the feelings of hunger or satiety, hence the quantities of food taking. Thermoregulation (all the mechanisms keeping the body temperature within normal limits) is controlled by the hypothalamus. The hypothalamus is also well-known for playing a more specific role in the emotional process. Its lateral part seems to be involved in such emotions as pleasure, rage, and its median part in aversion, displeasure and an uncontrolled tendency to laugh. First of all, the hypothalamus generates symptomatic manifestations of emotions and its role in generating affective states is only marginal. It therefore constitutes the emotional effector, causing and controlling the somatic and visceral reactions accompanying emotions. It is now clear that the limbic system exchanges numerous relationships with the hypothalamus, which co-ordinates the somatovegetative reactions underlying emotional states. Nevertheless, the limbic system is also in relation with associated areas in the cortex and especially with the prefrontal areas interfering in controlling emotions, in intentional role, in the intentional control of expressions of emotions and in the cognitive assessment of the emotional signification of complex social situations. These cortical areas are designated as being the place where mental and private experience of emotion is elaborated. This refers to Damasio's research work when he defined what he considered to be the final state of the emotional process, *feeling*.

3.3.2. The amygdala

This small-volume structure in the shape of an almond is located deep in the temporal lobe in its lower front part. The amygdala is the point of convergence of all sensory messages from specific associative areas such as vision, hearing, touch and olfaction. It has connections to and from the hippocampus, the septal nuclei of the prefrontal area and the back median nuclei of the thalamus. All those numerous and sophisticated connections give the amygdala a basic rôle in mediating as well as in controlling the main affective states.

The amygdala plays a basic role in the preservation of the human being, as it is the spot where danger is identified, resulting in fear and fright. If the amygdala is stimulated, a feeling of fear or anxiety can be generated with a maximum alert level inducing the individual to flee or to fight. In animals, experimental bilateral destruction of amygdalas brings about Klüver-Bucy's syndrome. On the other hand, deep brain stimulation of these structures generates violent crises of aggressiveness. In man, bilateral lesions of the amygdala lead to states of placidity and affective indifference.

3.3.3. The Septal Region

Phylogenetically, the septal region exists at a very early stage in the embryo and in the animal species; it is the first stage of the telencephalon. Anatomically, it is a narrow cortical area situated just before the front commissure and under the rostrum of the corpus callosum; it is very slightly raised on the median cortex; so it is the higher part of the "diagonal strip" above the para-olfactory cortex:

The septal region is connected with all primitive formations, whether limbic or hemispheric:

- each of the six following limbic rings has a foot in the septal region, the front commissure is the place where both septal regions meet,on the other hand, the septal region has reciprocal links with:

1. the olfactory tubercle through the diagonal strip
2. the paramedian nuclei of the hypothalamus behind the "final blade"

3. the amygdalian nucleus through the "ventral vegetative" fasciculus and through the final striatum
4. the nucleus accumbens (NAC) considered as ventral striatum
5. the innominate substance (Meynert) considered as ventral pallidum
6. the basal front cortex through the radiation of the rostrum of the corpus callosum

Interventricular Septum

It consists of two blades placed side by side, which are in fact the sharpened continuations of the median cortices going up to the corpus callosum; we can distinguish two different parts:

- the "septum lucidum": it is thin and forms the partition between the side ventricles
- the "septum verum": it is thick and rich in grey matter having its roots in the septal regions

The whole (septal regions + interventricular septum + front commissure) forms a fixed point which lies at the centre of the future developments of the limbic system and of the hemispheres. Stimulating these regions in animals results in a series of sexual manifestations, especially erection and ejaculation in males; these reactions are associated with preservation of the species. Stimulating the same regions in man does not bring about any sexual behaviour, but generally results subjective feelings of warmth and pleasure, often with sexual connotations.

3.3.4. The Frontal Lobes

The frontal lobes play a major role in the highest operation levels of human behaviour. These cortical regions are thought to be notably involved in social attitudes as well as in controlling, elaborating, regulating emotions, in adaptive behaviours and in a certain number of functions grouped under the heading of executive functions.

Although the initial definition of executive functions comes from cognitive psychology, the concept grew richer with data coming from clinical in relation with the functioning of prefrontal areas. These frontal functions, especially executive functions – both concepts do not overlap completely – are important for basic acquisitions in children. Dysfunction of these functions contributes to generating learning disorders (Denckla, 1996) but is by no means limited to that. Knowledge of the impact of frontal lobe lesions on certain social skills in adults had started with the Phineas Gage case in the late 19th century (Damasio, 1995). However, olfactory research work in the mid-20th century (Hebb, 1945) denied any damage to the superior cognitive functions following lesions; they were used to justify frontal lobectomies practiced on psychiatric patients and resulted years later in a series of research work on the unsuspected cognitive sequels of frontal lesions (Stuss et Benson, 1986). In fact, frontal lobes did not get the attention they are now given until the remarkable reflections of Luria (1973a) based on his neuropsychological assessments carried out on victims of WWII. Several researchers eventually attempted to find a solution to the puzzle of the frontal lobe from studies on patients with brain lesions and tried to draw up explanatory models of its functioning; the one that is mostly used today is Shallice (1982, 1988); his supervising attention system is largely inspired by the action control functions that Luria had attributed to frontal lobes. The frontal lobe can be divided into three parts: motor cortex, pre-motor cortex (or motor association area) and prefrontal cortex which includes all the non-motor areas of frontal lobes. Prefrontal lobe perturbations, known as frontal syndrome, are described following lesions in neuropsychology and in neuroscience. They are divided into three parts: a dorso-lateral face, an orbitary, ventral or inferior face and a median or internal face consisting of the cingular gyrus included in the limbic system. The prefrontal cortex, which virtually represents one third of the cortex mass, has multiple connections, the main ones with the motor system, the sensory neocortex and the limbic system. Indeed, the frontal lobes receive direct projections (most of which being doubled by reciprocal projections) from the temporal, parietal and occipital associative areas. The prefrontal cortex is also the only neocortical site to receive information passing through the limbic circuits and is linked through numerous connections to the limbic lobe (consisting of the cingular gyrus and the parahippocample gyrus), to the thalamus and the hypothalamus. So, frontal lobes can gain access to information about the viscero-endocrinian state, the motivational state and the emotional state of the individual. This is the reason why the prefrontal lobe has been considered to be an interface between cognition and emotion.

3.3.5. Emotions and Hemispheric Lateralisation

The complex management of emotions seems to be lateralised in the cerebral hemispheres in two ways. The left hemisphere is particularly involved in the intentional control of the expression of emotions, whereas the right hemisphere is specialised in the vegetative expression and the genesis of immediate emotions directly triggered by environment; it is also involved in the perceptive processing of emotions, i.a. in identifying expressions. A second set of data concerning the specialisation of the hemispheres in emotions has to do with the regulation of temper. It is believed that there is a superiority of the right hemisphere on negative emotions like sadness, anxiety and fright. So, pathologies of the minor hemisphere lead to indifference, agnosia, but also to semiology of delirium, lunacy and fantasising. On the contrary, the dominant hemisphere is supposed to play a major part in regulating positive emotions. In case of a lesion in the left hemisphere, the most frequently described pathologies are acute emotional reactions such as panic and disaster reactions with crying fits or depressive or aggressive attitudes with harassment or opposition behaviour.

4. The Mechanism of Fear

Fear and fright reactions that bring about defence behaviours (avoidance, aversion, anger) are probably innate and fall within the field of phylogenesis, corresponding to the famous basic programme discovered in the hypothalamus by Cannon and Bart. Fear and fright reactions do not appear at birth: a young baby is completely trusting and expects that his urges will be satisfied immediately – in accordance with the pleasure principle. Between seven and twelve months of age, the child begins to be afraid of strangers. Pressure circuits set up during this critical period characterised by mothering, feeding and the first footsteps. It means that the child gradually gains its independence and this enables him to adapt its defences to dangers. Initially, fear and fright are triggered by anything unusual or unknown. Indeed, as long as you do not really know, it is more cautious to be timid and then overcome your fear according to your own experience. It would even seem that certain fears are innate (archaic cerebrum and genetic memory) and that they are part of the genetic heritage: being afraid of insects, snakes, mice, of the dark, of heights, etc ... According to Jung, these innate protective reactions are part of the collective unconscious. Fear –and dealing with it – will then guide our experience and the way stimuli are going to shape the individual's history and man's future. The stage of absolute protection given by the mother is followed by the stages of parental upbringing with scolding, banning, warnings and punishment: so, emotions teach us how to live and survive in such surroundings. The biggest part of knowledge on fear and fright, emotions and memory derives from studies of classical conditioning of fear. This learning process is relatively easy to observe in laboratory conditions, as it is present in all animals, even the rat. In most models concerning fear and fright, pain is used as marker, as an unpleasant feeling likely to link a reaction of fear with the particular conditions of a traumatic experience.

In the same way, one experiment is sometimes enough to trigger fear reactions in the observed animal. Nevertheless, if the same stimuli are repeated without creating any pain, the reaction of fear diminishes: this is called the extinction or habituation phenomenon. So, the brain seems to control fear and fright reactions, but the emotional memory does not disappear. A reaction of conditioned fear can reappear spontaneously or during a stressful experience without any relationship with the stimulus, so referring to notions of uncontrollable and uncontrolled fright out of context.

Finally, a stressful experience can revive phobia-like phenomena in anxious people who had been ill but were apparently cured. This suggests that the emotional memory keeps traces of these phobias, which lay dormant but have not been erased by the medical treatment. In the same way, learning about the conditions under which this fear or fright occurred will eventually lead to restoring memories associated with this situation. The fear conditioning mechanism influences certain regions of the brain, which no longer distinguish stimuli in the same way. Joseph LeDoux already identified the cerebral circuit responsible for this conditioning in the 1980s.

5. Identifying Cerebral Structures Involved in Aversion Conditioning

Aversion conditioning is an experiment that can easily be carried out in a laboratory. It has been used for determining which neural circuits are implied in behaviours related with fear. Conditioned fear is the process by which a meaningless stimulus becomes associated with the sign of an impending danger. An example: if your neighbour's dog has already bitten you, you will probably be scared every time you have to go to his ground. You have merely associated your neighbour's trees and building with the painful biting of his dog. In a laboratory, conditioned fear experiments occur most often with a rat placed in a cage whose floor can yield slight electrical discharges. A sound is then sent out, immediately followed by a slight electric shock to the rat's paws. After a few associated sounds (conditional stimuli) and shocks (unconditional stimuli), the rat gets scared as soon as he hears the sound. The neutral stimulus (sound) has triggered conditioned fear. Conditioned fear can not only be initiated very quickly; it also has the advantage of lasting for a very long time. This kind of association is very strong and is not likely to be forgotten, which makes it possible to test it without worrying about the amount of time elapsed since it was learned. Another advantage of conditioned fear is that the phenomenon could be induced in practically all species, from the fly to the mollusc and from the fish to the ape. It seems to have been preserved in evolution and to play a basic role in the survival of species. But the most interesting points are that, first, the sensory system used for conditioning is often well-known and can be used as a starting-point to trace back the involved cerebral tracts; secondly, the behavioural fear response involves several well-known physiological modifications which can be measured (accelerated heart rate, higher rate of stress hormones in blood, etc.). We have to deal with the following problem: how can a new meaningless sound stimulus trigger a defensive behavioural response following some conditioned fear? Researchers have two firm starting-points to solve this problem: they know the starting point of the phenomenon (the auditory system and its connections within the brain) and the arriving point (the behavioural defence response with its visceral manifestations). So, they still had to find the connections linking inputs to outputs. Joseph LeDoux from New York University was one of the first researchers to have revived the scientific study of emotions through his experiments on conditioned fear. In a first series of experiments he first wondered which parts of the auditory system were essential to trigger conditioned fear. Lesions were first performed on the auditory cortex, where sounds were identified. But conditioned fear could still be induced in these animals. The region just before the cortex, the auditory thalamus, was then removed in certain rats. Unlike those whose cortex had been removed, they could no longer learn to experience conditioned fear The effect was the same in case of lesions at the subjacent station, the mesencephalon. So it became obvious that as far as conditioning was concerned, the auditory stimulus had to go to the thalamus. But where did it go then to trigger the emotional fear reaction? At the time, neuroanatomy handbooks just indicated the auditory cortex as output for the auditory thalamus. LeDoux and his colleagues then resorted to tracing techniques of neural tracts making it possible to visualise the paths followed by axons by injecting certain substances absorbed by neurones. Four subcortical regions receiving axons from the auditory thalamus were emphasised. A series of experiments in which each of these tracts was destroyed one after the other led to the discovery that the only one tract needed to create conditioned fear was the one leading to the amygdala. The discovery of this new subcortical path explained why auditory cortex lesions, which prevented the animal from identifying the sound accurately, did not eliminate conditioned fear: the neural tract from the thalamus to the amygdala merely bypassed the cortex. At the same time, another researcher, Bruce Kapp, had discovered a subregion of the amygdala, the central nucleus, which had connections with brainstem regions involved in controlling the heart rate and various responses of the vegetative nervous system. In the light of these various studies LeDoux suggested that these regions are the output of the amygdala causing the numerous visceral responses of conditioned fear. Shortly afterwards, a study of a lesion in the central nucleus showed that his intuition was right: the destruction of the central nucleus dramatically interfered with the behavioural response of conditioned fear. Thanks to lesion and tracing techniques, the basic wiring could be ascertained as well as the main cerebral structures involved in reactions of conditioned fear. Other studies eventually underlined the central role of the amygdala in fear emotion, independently of the nature of the sensory stimulus at the onset.

6. Identifying Cerebral Structures Involved in Context Fear Reactions

It is noteworthy that after a series of conditioning tests the animal reacts in a stereotyped way whenever it is put back into the experimentation cage: the rat keeps still as if it was paralysed with fear. This attitude of fear in relation to the context and not to the conditional stimulus probably represents the animal's reaction of protection in a dangerous environment. This context fear reaction is completely deleted in case of bilateral lesion of the hippocampus. More specifically, the back part of the hippocampus is necessary to learn the association between an aversion experience and the context. Interestingly enough, a lesion of the ventral hippocampus, which is strongly connected to the amygdala, inhibits learning and expressing aversion conditioning, in other words grasping that there is a link between an aversion stimulus (a shock) and a conditional stimulus (a tone).

7. The Circuit of Fear

Experimenting from targeted lesions in the brain of a conditioned rat, LeDoux was able to demonstrate that the sound that conditions fear does not need to be identified by the auditory cortex; it just has to be conveyed from the inner ear through the thalamus or the amygdalian nucleus. The destruction of the central nucleus of the amygdala (output towards the hypothalamus and the motor tracts) deletes the innate defence behaviour in relation with sound and the appropriate vegetative reactions. LeDoux then showed that there were two cerebral circuits to access to the amygdalian nuclei. This explains why they react differently according to the level at which they interpret the visual or sound stimulus: a quick but inaccurate direct circuit from the thalamus and an accurate but slow indirect circuit passing through the auditory and visual cortex.

Coming back to fright, let us take the example of a solitary visitor in a haunted house or one reputed as such. He hears moaning so he jumps with fright and stops – this is an animal's first quick reaction to potential danger. Simultaneously, the auditory cortex elaborates an analysis that will confirm or infirm the threat; if it identifies a creaking door, it will defuse the original reaction of fear and fright. Learning about this experience is taken over by activating neurotransmittors such as glutamate, which induces long-term potentialisation in the post-synaptic receptors of the amygdala. This reinforced synaptic connection represents the biological link of the conditional association between the stimulus and the reaction of fear and fright. Blocking these amygdalian receptors inhibits conditioning.

There are two types of neurones reacting to sound stimuli: some get used to them and others still react. Those that get used to stimuli finally no longer react to repeated sounds; they would be used to detect unusual sounds and enable the amygdalian nuclei to ignore stimuli that have got familiar. On the contrary, a shock prevents cells from getting used: they do not ignore – they react.

8. THE NEUROBIOLOGY OF FEAR

1. Afferent Nervous Signal

The main nervous stimuli received by our brain in case of a reaction of fright are visual, auditory, tactile and cognitive stimuli; they vary extremely from one person to another. The brain is then going to achieve a summation of the received information in the form of action potentials; it is worth noting that cognitive stimuli play a major role, as motivation is often the releasing factor.

2. Neural Integration And Efferent Nervous Message

Once the summation of the various stimuli and motivations has been carried out, you decide to yield to the stimulus even if you are still somewhat apprehensive. From a physiological point of view, the summation of information afferent to your cortex - plus some new stimuli (the most famous ones being physical stimuli) – delivers a message (understand the efferent action potential) indicating an instinctive defence reflex to danger. This action potential originating from the cortex is then conveyed all along the spinal cord to reach two endocrine glands located on the kidneys: the medulla-adrenal glands.

3. Transforming the Nervous Signal into A Hormonal Signal

Under the pressure of the action potential, the gland secretes a hormone, adrenaline, which is released in blood. This hormone has a whole range of physiological effects on numerous effectors, among others: the heart (accelerated heart rate) and blood vessels (vasoconstriction, hence increased blood pressure). The effects of adrenaline are to be felt very easily; this is the reason why in everyday life we speak of "an adrenaline rush" occurring after a strong emotion.

4. Describing Adrenaline

Adrenaline is a hormone secreted by the medulla-adrenal glands. It is a amina acid, so a definite gene codes. Adrenaline has far-reaching effects, the major ones being that it adheres to heart cells receptors and to the receptors of cells lining blood vessel walls.

5. Retrocontrol Action - Notion of a Regulated Biological System

When released in blood adrenaline causes major physiological changes (accelerated heart rate and vasoconstriction), but the adrenaline content of blood is also detected by the brain through specific membrane receptors. If we intend to overcome our fear, adrenaline can be deleted or recycled (once it has disappeared from blood circulation, it will no longer act on effectors). Repression of fear is caused by a nervous signal sent by the hypothalamus (part of the encephalon located beneath the cortex, in the lateral of the third ventricule) which will trigger the secretion of proteins aimed either at recycling or destroying adrenaline. This secretion takes place in the endocrine glands. We can therefore speak of control action and of a regulated biological system.

9. Fear, Fright and Biology: A Summary

This neurobiological description is very simplified, as mechanisms of fear can not only be explained through the action of adrenaline; other hormones come into play and the role of the nervous system is not only to release secretions (it is responsible for reflexes like shutting your eyes, curling up, attempting to scream or run away, etc...). In the case of a fear or fright reaction, adrenaline is identified as "a reward" by the hypothalamic receptors, which activates the so-called reward mechanism. It is worth mentioning that fear is a physiological phenomenon bringing into play two major "communication systems" (the neural one and the hormonal one). Reactions occur instinctively (stimuli – central nervous system – effectors) and fear regulation is then carried out using cognition.

9.1. At The Neuro-Anatomic Level

Three regions of the brain hierarchically take part in the making of fear:

1. *The prefrontal cortex* assesses danger thanks to memories, events or emotions associated with previous experiences ; it also controls conditioned reactions using a learning method by extinction.
2. *The amygdalian nuclei* of the limbic system play a role in triggering conditioned reactions of fear.
3. *The hypothalamus* receives internal and external stress signals and triggers motor and visceral alarm reactions to the detected threats. The hypothalamus also acts through hormones. It secretes a hormone, CRF (corticotropin releasing factor), which stimulates the pituitary gland, located under the hypothalamus, which in turn releases a second hormone, the ACTH (adrenocorticotropic hormone). Once it has been released into blood circulation, ACTH stimulates the adrenal glands, which in turn release cortisol, a third hormone preparing the body to defend itself: the defence consists in increasing the quantity of energy delivered to the heart, to the brain and to the skeletal muscles. ACTH and cortisol also have a direct effect on the brain by increasing alert and motivation reactions and by stimulating the hippocampus, and thus memory processes. There is a wide range of fear symptoms. They include: perspiring, feeling nervous, trembling, quivering, feeling of suffocation, breathlessness, quick or evasive looks, quick breathing, having a lump in the throat, having tensed muscles, cramps, diarrhoea, vomiting, urinating, being cold, having gooseflesh or heartburn. All these symptoms clearly indicate that fear and fright are not merely "cortical" and that the body as a whole sympathises and reacts to this

emotion. On the other hand, an attack of the central amygdala targets impedes fear expression; an attack of the hypothalamus brings about higher blood pressure; an attack of the Sylvius aqueduct grey matter does not cause corticals activation; an attack of the final stria nuclei hinders the secretion of the stress hormone through the hypothalamohypophyseal axis.

9.2. Behaviour Circuits

So, fear and fright are the starting-point triggering a behaviour model. In 1922, Kleist had stressed the importance of the striatum and the other basal nuclei as well as their links with the prefrontal cortex as a mediator of behaviour. Nauta traced links between these circuits and the limbic system in 1986. Then, from 1986 to 1990, Alexander established the three parallel circuits controlling behaviour independently: we have to do with retroactive loops which start from distinct parts of the frontal lobe, follow parallel but individual ways and connect successively to the putamen, the pallidum and the thalamus before returning to the cortical region from where they started.

- **The first circuit**, known as the cingular frontal circuit, is responsible for initiative. Its destruction leads, to variable extent, to a lack of interest such as apathy, a loss of initiative for speaking (mutism) and for voluntary movement (akinesia) as well as affective indifference or even a mental void.
- **The second circuit**, known as the orbito-frontal circuit, is responsible for inhibiting drives. Any dysfunction of this system whose role is to suppress stimulation from the outside world or from internal needs brings about antisocial behaviour. Dysfunction in this orbito-frontal circuit yields a full range of impulsion control disorders such as obsessive compulsive disorders, anorexia, bulimia, drug addiction, pathological gambling or shopping, kleptomania, pyromania, exhibitionism, voyeurism and violence.
- **The third circuit** has an executive function. It supervises planning, sequence organisation and the performance of adaptation strategies. It is responsible for flexibility, adaptation efficiency and imagination to solve a problem. It adds a rational element in emotions, especially in fear and fright. Until recently decision-making was considered to be a superior cognitive function based on an objective and "rational" analysis of the outside world. However, in the light of research work published over the past decades, we have to admit that an animal bases its decisions not only on external information but also on its momentary internal state and on past experience stored in its memory, which gives him an internal reference. These (controllable or controlled) internal references enable the animal to choose what is right or wrong in its environment. It would indeed have been far too difficult, too time-consuming and "neural space-consuming" for the nervous system to store all possibilities and the countless models of all possible options. So, the decisionmaking space, at least in animals, is rather small because of the internal state of the animal. This also applies to its memory, which gives values to common options. So, fear and fright fully illustrate the fact that we decide with "our guts", as the saying goes.

10. Fear and Fright: Some Clinical Extensions

10.1. Fear, Fright and Terror During Sleep

Unlike dyssomnias, parasomnias do not imply abnormal waking-sleeping mechanisms. They essentially consist in activating the physiological and neurological systems occurring at various stages of sleep.

Nightmares

Repeated occurrence of frightening dreams causing complete waking up with a feeling of failure, discomfort or impending physical danger accompanied by a persisting sensation of fear or anxiety. Events are real (rare) or not. Nightmares occur more frequently during the second part of the night and during REM sleep. Difficulties to go back to sleep.

Associated Disorders

Slight neurovegetative activity (sudation, tachycardia, etc...); there are generally no associated movements (inhibition during REM sleep). Symptoms of depression and anxiety.

Connectivity Examination

Sudden waking up during REM sleep. Increased heart rate or respiratory frequency. In cases of post-traumatic syndrome, nightmares during stage 2. Prevalence: 10 to 50% of children aged 3-5 years; up to 50% of the population suffers from occasional nightmares. Nightmares often start between 3 and 6 years of age and tend to disappear as people get older.

Nightmares should not be mistaken for night terrors, which generally occur during the first third of the night (stages 3 and 4); in this case, no traces are kept in memory (except for a few non-narrative isolated images). Moreover, the person wakes up only partially and there is amnesia of the events when he/she wakes up in the morning. The same applies to fits of panic.

Night Terrors

Sudden waking up starting with a cry of terror or tears. The person sits up. It occurs in the first third of the night and lasts from one to ten minutes (once a night). Neurovegetative activation and behavioural manifestations of intense fear. Difficulties to wake up and to get comforted (the person is disorientated for a few minutes). No narrative dream activity. Amnesia when waking up.

Associated Disorders

Howling, yelling, crying, incoherent vocalisation. Elaborate motor activity (getting up, punching, etc...). In adults, these disorders correspond to generalised anxiety, post-traumatic syndromes, dependent personality disorders, and a schizoid personality, borderline.

Connectivity Examination

Occurs at stages 3 – 4. EEG activity high-voltage delta at the onset. Theta or alpha activity during the episode. Increased muscular tonus. Accelerated heart rate (2 or 3 times as much as usually). Sometimes sudden waking up during deep sleep. Prevalence: 1 to 6% in children and less than 1 % in adults. Starts in children between 4 and 12 years of age and disappears when they become teenagers. Starts in adults between 20 and 30 years with a chronic evolution. Night terrors should not be mixed up with convulsive crises, which occur above all during transitions from waking to sleep (incontinence and tonico-clonic movements + Δ EEG) and with panic disorders causing the person to wake up quickly, completely and without confusion (same symptoms as for day panic disorders). The description of these sleeping disorders helps us to understand that fear, fright and terror are not limited to our conscious and unconscious diurnal life; even in periods where the brain functions differently (and this includes sleeping stages, especially REM sleep), the various neural networks and beings as a whole are likely to experience full frights in their bodies and heads.

10.2. Fear, Fright and the Epileptic Model

SEEG and some clinical situations in epileptology enable us to visualise "live" discharge phenomena in different structures predefined when placing ventricular electrodes. What emerges from these analyses when visualising pre-, per- and postictal epilectic phenomena is that seizures in mnesial structures affecting the amygdala, the temporal lobe and the hippocampus lead to compulsive behaviours, to fear and fright. In the same way, circuits including the ventral and pre-ventral part of the frontal lobes seem to be involved in generating emotional manifestations of fear and fright. In their article *"Fear, anger and compulsive behavior during seizure: involvement of large scale fronto-temporal neural networks"* Bartolomeil and colleagues discussed the various networks potentially associated and involved in emotional behaviours during a seizure. Seizure-related, abnormal affective and gestural behaviour may involve some of the same processes as those underlying non-pathological behaviour, but their mechanisms remain largely unknown. In this report, we studied a patient whose seizures initially involved the medial temporal region before involving the frontal cortex. Seizure semiology of the second part of the seizure included marked emotional disturbances (dominated by intense fear and anger) and compulsive behaviour to bite into something. This patient underwent presurgical evaluation including intracerebral electroencephalographic recordings (SEEG, stereoelectroencephalography). In addition to SEEG examination, we used coherence analysis of signals as a means of studying functional coupling between different regions of the brain. Two seizures were studied. Coherence values from different periods of interest were compared to identify the neural structures involved at the onset of seizure activity as well as during the emotional behavioral changes. They conclude that a first network of neural structures was identified within the right front temporal regions (amygdala, temporal pole, hippocampus, and temporal neocortex). At the time of intense affective and compulsive changes, and by comparison with the first ictal period, a second network was identified characterised by significant functional coupling between the amygdala, the orbito-frontal structures and the frontal opercular region, while a decrease in functional coupling between these regions and the dorsolateral region and the cingular gyrus was apparent.

11. Conclusion

This study shows that the emergence of an intense affective and behavioural state during a temporal lobe seizure could be related to the involvement of a network of structures including the front temporal lobe and the orbito-frontal cortex. The decrease of coupling between these regions and the lateral prefrontal and cingular regions could also participate in these phenomena. This type of observations leaves a clear field to a better understanding of the complex mechanisms involved in generating an emotion – more specifically fright – by implying numerous networks including the temporal and orbito-frontal lobes.

11.1. Fear and Fright: The Deep Brain Stimulation (DBS) Implantation Model

Another theoretical model is likely to bring information on the structures involved in emotions by means of thalamic or subthalamic intracranial electrodes implantations for the treatment of Parkinson's disease.

In his article *"Transient acute depression induced by DBS"*, Bejjani emphasises the fact that continuous high-frequency stimulation in certain regions of the brain can induce "emotional" behaviours. Continuous high-frequency stimulation of the basal ganglia was recently introduced for the treatment of patients with advanced Parkinson's disease. This treatment seems to be most effective when the electrodes are placed in the subthalamic nuclei. We describe here the results of detailed studies of the induction of major, reversible depression in this woman. A 65-year-old right-handed woman with a 30-year history of Parkinson's disease, who had severe rigidity, severe akinesia, and moderate tremor while resting, despite treatment with 900 mg of levodopa, 2.5 mg of pergolide, and 3 to 5 mg of lorazepam daily. Disabling dyskinesias induced by levodopa led to bilateral implantation of electrodes in the region of the subthalamic nuclei for stimulation therapy. She had no history of psychiatric disorders or depression, even after the onset of Parkinson's disease, nor mood fluctuations while receiving levodopa. The quadripolar electrodes implanted under stereotactic guidance were connected by a cable under the scalp extending to a programmable pulse generator placed under the skin in the subclavicular area, like a cardiac pacemaker. Each electrode had four contacts numbered 0 to 3 from bottom to top, over a length of 7.5 mm, permitting a choice of the most effective sites of stimulation in the target region.

To identify the optimal site, the effect of stimulation through each of the four contacts of each electrode was evaluated 10 days after surgery and 12 hours after the most recent dose of levodopa, according to our standardized protocol. During this postoperative evaluation, the patient's face expressed profound sadness within five seconds after a continuous monopolar 2.4-V rectangular current with a pulse width of 60 µsec and a frequency of 130 Hz was delivered for seven minutes through contact 0 of the electrode implanted on the left. Although still alert, the patient leaned to the right, started to cry, and verbally communicated feelings of sadness, guilt, uselessness, and hopelessness such as "I'm falling down in my head, I no longer wish to live, to see anything, hear anything, feel anything. . . .". When asked why she was crying and if she felt pain, she responded: "No, I'm fed up with life, I've had enough. . . . I don't want to live any more, I'm disgusted with life. . . . Everything is useless, always feeling worthless, I'm scared in this world." When asked why she was sad, she replied: "I'm tired. I want to hide in a corner. . . . I'm crying over myself, of course. . . . I'm hopeless, why am I bothering you. . . ." She had no hallucinations, nor were there any changes in her motor or cognitive symptoms of Parkinson's disease. The depression disappeared less than 90 seconds after stimulation was stopped. For the next five minutes the patient was in a slightly hypomanic state, and she laughed and joked with the examiner, playfully pulling his tie. She recalled the entire episode. Márcio L.S. Bezerra also writes in his article *"Transient Acute Depression Induced by High-Frequency Deep-Brain Stimulation"*: Bejjani et al. reported the induction of transient acute depression by stimulation of the left subthalamic nucleus in a woman with Parkinson's disease. We have found that pallidotomy may also cause depression in patients with this disease. Among 41 patients (25 men and 16 women; mean age at operation, 60 years) with severe, chronic Parkinson's disease, 17 underwent left-sided pallidotomy, 13 right-sided pallidotomy, and 11 bilateral pallidotomy. All the patients improved after surgery. Persistent major depression, as defined by the *Diagnostic and Statistical Manual of Mental Disorders,* developed immediately after the surgical procedure in five of these patients, all of whom had undergone left-sided pallidotomy. The 5 patients did not differ from the other 36 patients with regard to sex or age, duration of Parkinsonian symptoms, severity of symptoms as assessed by ‰Te Unified Parkinson's Disease Rating Scale, or extent of improvement after pallidotomy. They were treated with a selective serotonin-reuptake inhibitor and improved markedly. These findings point to the pivotal role played by the basal ganglia in mood disorders and to the functional asymmetry of the brain. These two articles show us that through DBS techniques we actually influence structures essential to generate emotions but also that a better understanding of the diffusion models of electrical fields emitted in a given environment is unavoidable to determine the "type of action" " we can have through these treatments i.a. on neural networks responsible for emotions, fear and perhaps fright...

11.2. Emotions, Fear, Fright and the Vestibular System

In virtually all cases, a vestibular neuritis, a short-, middle- or long-lived pathology of the Ménière type generates a vast vertigo syndrome associated, broadly speaking, with a vagal malaise. What is most important is the fact that these symptomes are very often associated with an emotional behaviour closely connected with fear, panic or anxiety. It is worth mentioning that, if symptoms are not identified straightaway as "slight", the patient will in a certain number of cases develop eventual phobia behaviours, fits of panic often associated with loss of control and impending death. This association – real-life experience plus memories plus emotions (possibly frights) – is an interesting approach in the debate about the balance between the brain, the body and memories, as far as the management and understanding of fear and emotions are concerned.

12. Discussion

Amygdalian nuclei certainly play a major role in emotional behaviour, but experiments on rodents (LeDoux) have shown the structure of the various amygdalian nuclei and their role in learning fear and in restoring memories associated to fear. The lateral nucleus receives information from the sensory regions of the brain and passes on these signals to the baso-lateral, basal accessory and central nucleus. The central nucleus is connected to the brainstem, which triggers changes of the various physiological parameters. Thus, fear conditioning causes the formation of emotional memories in various animals. Once this memory associated with fear exits, it persists and we can often witness behavioural changes towards stimuli associated with fear, but the emotional memory is never eliminated - even when the emotional reaction is under control. The fact that there is some similarity in the results obtained in various species indicates that the cerebral circuits followed in this type of learning are the same along the phylogenesis. Locating an essential mechanism of emotional memory in the amygdalian circuit is useful in some respects. The amygdalian nucleus is a major site of learning because of its central position between sensory inputs and effector outputs. Every tract coming into the amygdalian nuclei brings in specific information. Circuits having their origin in the sensory thalamus only give a rough perception of the outside world, but they are very quick and contain only one neural relay. On the contrary, cortical circuits give accurate and detailed representations of the outside world enabling us to identify an object as soon as we see or hear it. These circuits, going from the thalamus to the sensory cortex sensory, then to the amygdalain nucleus include several neural relays. Each link in the chain slows down treatment. So, in the case of emotional learning, it is because of time pressure that there are two ways, a cortical way and a subcortical way. Both animals and human beings need some rough-and-ready reaction mechanism: so, the thalamus activates cortex and amygdalian nuclei practically at the same time, which brings about emotional reactions in amygdalian nuclei before identification of what we feel or the stimulus we react to. Emotional learning and all memories are stored and restored in parallel and are combined with our conscious experience, which does not mean at all that we have conscious and direct access to the emotional memory. This rather means that we have access to its consequences. Emotional memory systems with early developments are supposed to store unconscious memories of these events; this explains why an early trauma could disturb a person's mental and behavioural functions through unconscious mechanisms. Fear and fright are therefore a subjective alert state triggered by the cerebral systems reacting to danger. Conscious fear goes along with a physical reaction only in organisms with sufficiently developed neural mechanisms. Human beings may not be the only ones to experience fear or fright, however consciousness is essential to subjective emotional states.

13. Conclusions

Fear and fright are archaic functions leading to survival of primitive animals. These emotions have steadily kept evolving and they have even guided evolution while retaining its most efficient mechanisms. Alarm reactions, aggressive and consuming drives (hunger and pleasure), induction to pleasure, fear and fright are kept in the hypothalamus. All these data enable the limbic system (the amygdalian nucleus) to mark our learning by associations, by linking these informations to the rewarding or unpleasant effects of occurrences, thus allowing the selection of reinforcement behaviour (motivation) or avoidance behaviour (aversion).

Emotions, including fear and fright, enrich individual memory with experience that enables innate reactions to adapt simply, flexibly and efficiently to multisensory stimuli. Thanks to the expansion of the cerebral cortex the range of emotion expressions has got morý diverse and became a language controlling social life and co-operation as well as integration within or between species. Conscious and unconscious management of emotions turned into a decision-making system aimed at ruling behaviours of the highest levels. By choosing the high-capacity prefrontal cortex in direct relation with the outside world and our inner world, it enables us to assess in the form of personal impressions the future consequences of our powers of reasoning and our adaptation to exceptional situations. The combination of automatic (even archaic) vital functions – including fear and fright – and of modulation, memorisation, decision-making and expectation enables us to adapt to our environment and so, to continue evolving. Emotions, broadly speaking, allow us to code the world and to gain access to a non-verbal interpersonal language present in most species. The combination of non-verbal and verbal language contributes to the advancement of our thinking skills by including phenomena like intuition, reasoning, abstraction, analysis and synthesis. In this way, fear and fright, which are an integral part of emotions and the emotional language, construct and shape our personality and our behavioural attitudes so that we can go on evolving within our species in the world around us.

It should also ne noted that fear, fright and anxiety are notions that should not be mixed up. Anxiety is an emotion that is different from fear or fright. Anxiety is unfounded, it stimulates the attention paid to the outside world and it often intensifies senses and pain perception. Nowadays dangerous and frightening situations in terms of survival of species and its offspring are rather rare in comparison with prehistoric times or the Reign of Terror during the French Revolution. However the existential circumstances of our society are creating new situations of fear and fright (people are afraid of nuclear disaster, of a world war, of AIDS). On the contrary, fear and fright focus on accurate situations and lead to act either automatically or after planning. Fear and fright must be a heritage of the past, something left over from our most distant ancestors as through them they got aware of situations of danger (alarm, defence, escape or pursuit - according to situations in which these vital emotions enabled them, e.g. cave men, to survive in spite of danger). It may be that nowadays men as we are fear what our ancestors dreaded. In the real-life experience of a given human being, we often forget the circumstances that have imprinted this fright or terror in body and brain. So a memory can resurface years after a traumatic event without it being possible to determine when the occurrence actually started and what its mnesic foothold was. This type of amnesia could be linked to the fact that under stress the hippocampus is less efficient towards the amygdalian complex, which is stimulated by stress while strengthening fear and fright conditioning. In these situations, fear and fright can be unconsciously engraved into cerebral structures, on a long-term basis and without any control.

14. A Final Remark: The Freud's Position

What sort of man are we talking about? Is fear experienced by man towards reality something normal, "natural", or does it result from some particular upbringing that has accustomed him to fright? According to Freud, only the man brought up to beliefs since his early days will necessarily continue to feel a need to believe: he was "instilled the sweet and bitter poison" and he can no longer do without it, he becomes an addict, religion becomes a kind of drug or tranquilliser and it will "daze the neurosis it has initiated at the beginning."

15. Ackowledgments

We would like to acknowledge Professor P. Deltenre, X and Marie Bronchart for their help in the writing of this chapter.

16. References

Acierno, R., Rheingold, A.A., Resnick, H.S. and Kilpatrick, D.G., Predictors of fear of crime in older adults, *J. Anxiety Disord,* 18 (2004) 385-96.

Adolphs,R et al.*neurosc.* (2000) 20:2685

Adolphs, R., Neural systems for recognizing emotions in humans. In M.K. Hauser, M. (Ed.), *Neural mechanisms of cimmunication,* MIT Press, Cambridge, MA, 1999, pp. 187-212.

Adolphs, R., Damasio, H., Tranel, D., Cooper, G. and Damasio, A.R., A role for somatosensory cortices in the visual recognition of emotion as revealed by three-dimensional lesion mapping, *J. Neurosci,* 20 (2000) 2683-90.

Adolphs, R., Tranel, D. and Damasio, A.R., Dissociable neural systems for recognizing emotions, *Brain Cogn,* 52 (2003) 61-9.

Adolphs, R., Tranel, D., Damasio, H. and Damasio, A.R., Fear and the human amygdala, *J. Neurosci,* 15 (1995) 5879-91.

Alexander, D.A., Klein, S., Gray, N.M., Dewar, I.G. and Eagles, J.M., Suicide by patients: questionnaire study of its effect on consultant psychiatrists, *Bmj,* 320 (2000) 1571-4.

Bard, K.A., Development of emotional expressions in chimpanzees (Pan troglodytes), *Ann. N. Y. Acad. Sci,* 1000 (2003) 88-90.

Bartolomeil, F., Guye, M., Wendling, F., Gavaret, M., Regis, J. and Chauvel, P., Fear, anger and compulsive behavior during seizure: involvement of large scale fronto-temporal neural networks, *Epileptic Disord,* 4 (2002) 235-41.

Bejjani, B.P., Damier, P., Arnulf, I., Thivard, L., Bonnet, A.M., Dormont, D., Cornu, P., Pidoux, B., Samson, Y. and Agid, Y., Transient acute depression induced by high-frequency deep-brain stimulation, *N. Engl. J. Med,* 340 (1999) 1476-80.

Bezerra, M.L., Martinez, J.V. and Nasser, J.A., Transient acute depression induced by high-frequency deep-brain stimulation, *N. Engl. J. Med,* 341 (1999) 1003; author reply 1004.

Blair, R.J., Morris, J.S., Frith, C.D., Perrett, D.I. and Dolan, R.J., Dissociable neural responses to facial expressions of sadness and anger, *Brain,* 122 (Pt 5) (1999) 883-93.

Cannon, W.B., The James-Lange theory of emotions: a critical examination and an alternative theory. By Walter B. Cannon, 1927, *Am. J. Psychol,* 100 (1987) 567-86.

Damasio, A., Feelings of emotion and the self, *Ann. N. Y. Acad. Sci,* 1001 (2003) 253-61.

Damasio, A., Fundamental feelings, *Nature,* 413 (2001) 781.

Damasio, A.R., Descartes' error and the future of human life, *Sci. Am,* 271 (1994) 144.

Damasio, A.R., Descartes's error: emotion, reason, and the human brain, *Grosset/Putman,* 1994.

Damasio, A.R., Emotion in the perspective of an integrated nervous system, *Brain Res. Brain Res. Rev,* 26 (1998) 83-6.

Damasio, A.R., Neuropsychology. Towards a neuropathology of emotion and mood, *Nature,* 386 (1997) 769-70.

Damasio, A.R., Grabowski, T.J., Bechara, A., Damasio, H., Ponto, L.L., Parvizi, J. and Hichwa, R.D., Subcortical and cortical brain activity during the feeling of self-generated emotions, *Nat. Neurosci,* 3 (2000) 1049-56.

Denckla, M.B., Biological correlates of learning and attention: what is relevant to learning disability and attention-deficit hyperactivity disorder?, *J. Dev. Behav. Pediatr,* 17 (1996) 114-9.

Denckla, M.B., The neuropsychology of social-emotional learning disabilities, *Arch. Neurol,* 40 (1983) 461-2.

Ekman, P., Darwin, deception, and facial expression, *Ann. N. Y. Acad. Sci,* 1000 (2003) 205-21.

Ekman, P., Emotions inside out. 130 Years after Darwin's "The Expression of the Emotions in Man and Animal", *Ann. N. Y. Acad. Sci,* 1000 (2003) 1-6.

Ekman, P., Facial expression and emotion, *Am. Psychol,* 48 (1993) 384-92.

Ekman, P., Facial expressions of emotion: an old controversy and new findings, Philos. Trans. R. Soc. Lond. B. *Biol. Sci,* 335 (1992) 63-9.

Ford, R.E., Alexander, M. and Lester, D., Fear of death of those in a high stress occupation, *Psychol. Rep,* 29 (1971) 502.

Gall, M.D., The relationship between masculinity-femininity and manifest anxiety, *J. Clin. Psychol,* 25 (1969) 294-5.

Hebb, A.L., Zacharko, R.M., Dominguez, H., Laforest, S., Gauthier, M., Levac, C. and Drolet, G., Changes in brain cholecystokinin and anxiety-like behavior following exposure of mice to predator odor, *Neuroscience,* 116 (2003) 539-51.

Heller, W., Neuropsychological mechanisms of individual differences in emotion, personality, and arousal, *Neuropsychology,* 7 (1993) 476-489.

Herrick, J.B., Fear among consumers, *J. Am. Vet. Med. Assoc,* 204 (1994) 1874-5.

Kleist, K., Brain and psyche, *J. Nerv. Ment. Dis,* 116 (1952) 776-82.

LeDoux, j. In m. Gazzanig (Ed.), The Congnitive Neurosciences, MIT Press, Cambridge, MA, 1995, pp. 1049-1061.

LeDoux, J., The emotional brain, fear, and the amygdala, *Cell Mol. Neurobiol,* 23 (2003) 727-38.

LeDoux, J., Fear and the brain: where have we been, and where are we going?, *Biol. Psychiatry,* 44 (1998) 1229-38.

LeDoux, J.E., Emotion circuits in the brain, *Annu. Rev. Neurosci,* 23 (2000) 155-84.

Luria, R.E., Relationship between mood and digit-symbol performance in hospitalized patients with functional psychiatric disorders, *Psychol. Med,* 4 (1974) 454-9.

Luria, R.E., The validity and reliability of the visual analogue mood scale, *J. Psychiatr. Res,* 12 (1975) 51-7.

MacLean, P.D., Cerebral evolution and emotional processes: new findings on the striatal complex, *Ann. N. Y. Acad. Sci,* 193 (1972) 137-49.

Meltzoff, A.N., Perception, action, and cognition in early infancy, *Ann. Pediatr.* (Paris), 32 (1985) 63-77.

Meltzoff, A.N. and Moore, M.K., Imitation of facial and manual gestures by human neonates, *Science,* 198 (1977) 74-8.

Meltzoff, A.N. and Moore, M.K., Interpreting "imitative" responses in early infancy, *Science,* 205 (1979) 217-9.

Meltzoff, A.N. and Moore, M.K., Newborn infants imitate adult facial gestures, *Child. Dev,* 54 (1983) 702-9.

Monod-Broca, P., [Paul Broca: 1824-1880], *Ann. Chir,* 126 (2001) 801-7.

Moss, H. and Damasio, A.R., Emotion, cognition, and the human brain, *Ann. N. Y. Acad.* Sci, 935 (2001) 98-100.

Papez, J.W., A proposed mechanism of emotion. 1937, *J. Neuropsychiatry Clin. Neurosci,* 7 (1995) 103-12.

Rosenberg, M., [140th anniversary of the death of Franz Joseph Gall], *Psychiatr. Neurol. Med. Psychol.* (Leipz), 21 (1969) 357-8.

Russell, C.L., Bard, K.A. and Adamson, L.B., Social referencing by young chimpanzees (Pan troglodytes), *J. Comp. Psychol,* 111 (1997) 185-93.

Shallice, T., Functional imaging and neuropsychology findings: how can they be linked?, Neuroimage, 20 *Suppl.* 1 (2003) S146-54.

Shallice, T., 'Theory of mind' and the prefrontal cortex, *Brain,* 124 (2001) 247-8.

Stuss, D.T. and Benson, D.F., Neuropsychological studies of the frontal lobes, *Psychol. Bull,* 95 (1984) 3-28.

Wade, N.J., Erasmus Darwin (1731-1802), *Perception,* 31 (2002) 643-50.

Wyplosz, J., [Paul Broca: the protohistory of neurosurgery], *Rev. Prat,* 53 (2003) 937-40.

In: Fear in Cognitive Neuroscience
Editor: Salvatore Campanella, pp. 35-61

ISBN: 1-59454-502-2

Chapter 3

FEARFUL FACE PROCESSING IN ANXIETY

Céline Douilliez and Pierre Philippot
University of Louvain at Louvain-la-Neuve, Belgium

INTRODUCTION

From an evolutionary perspective, fear in one of the most relevant emotions for the survival of species. Fear enables a rapid detection of threat in the environment and prepares the organism to respond efficiently to the threat. Among potentially threatening stimuli, the face is particularly relevant. A wealth of research shows that humans have an innate ability to processes faces. Further, facial expression has a central signal value in social interactions as it reflects the behavioural intentions of the expresser.

If healthy individuals are able to rapidly detect and decode threatening facial expression and are biologically prepared to it, the role played by facial expression processing is particularly central for those suffering from emotional disorder. The aim of the present chapter is to review empirical studies and theoretical work relevant to the processing of nonverbal threatening signals in the etiology and the maintenance of anxiety.

We will first explore core facets of the normal processing of emotional facial expression regardless of their valence. A cognitive model of emotion will be presented as theoretical framework articulating different cognitive regulation processes. Then, we will present cognitive models of anxiety which postulate that biases in the processing of threatening stimuli are involved in the maintenance of anxiety disorders. Then, we will turn to empirical evidences of cognitive biases in anxiety, examining successively attentional biases, evaluative deficit and biases in facial decoding and memory biases for threatening faces in anxiety. We will conclude by integrating these different aspects, examining their clinical implications, and suggesting future directions for research.

The Processing of Emotional Facial Expression

In this section, we will explore different facets of the normal processing of emotional facial expression in general and of threatening facial expression in particular. Before reviewing data on facial expression decoding and emotional responses to threatening facial expression, we will overview data about the universality of facial expression of emotion.

Facial Expression of Emotion

According to the Darwin's evolutionary theory, facial movements have been selected by evolutionary processes because of their adaptive functions. Their main function would be to serve intra- and extra-species communication and regulation. Following this perspective, Ekman (1971) has proposed that there are innate "affect programs" linking "each primary emotion to a distinctive patterned set of neural impulses to the facial muscles" (Ekman, 1971, p.216). According to this theory, the number of so-called "primary" or "fundamental" or "basic" emotions is limited to a set of 7 emotions: happiness, sadness, fear, anger, surprise, disgust, and contempt. In addition to these basic emotions, Ekman and Friesen (1978) has proposed the existence of emotional "blends" occurring when more than one affect program are concurrently activated.

Recently, Ekman (1999) synthesized a series of characteristics that signs "basic emotions". Basic emotions would be universal distinctive signals that inform individuals on what is occurring for the person feeling the specific emotion: the specific antecedents and consequences and the internal state. Basic emotion would have distinctive universal antecedents, that is specific emotion would occur in specific situation, characterized by common features. Further, these antecedents would be similar across cultures. They also have distinctive patterns of autonomic nervous system activity and of regional brain activity. These patterns prepare the organism to respond specifically to a given emotional stimulus.

According to these characteristics, fear is one of the basic emotions. Fear is a universal distinctive signal. All over the world, a fear expression is interpreted as a response to something threatening in the environment and as indicating an urge to escape from the situation. Fear has also universal antecedents. For example, physical (e.g. facing a bear or a very angry person) or psychological harm (e.g. speaking in front of a large audience) elicit fear. Finally, there are evidences that fear differs from others emotions on several physiological responses (Stemmler, 2004). Different emotion eliciting tasks have been used to evidence differential pattern of physiological response. For example, in the directed facial action task, subjects are instructed to contract facial muscles in order to produce an emotional configuration. In the relieved emotions task, subjects have to relive emotional memories (for a review, see Levenson, 1992). These studies have evidenced larger heart rate acceleration for fear as compared to disgust and joy, and greater skin conductance response as compared to joy, and lower diastolic blood pressure, cooler surface temperatures, greater vasoconstriction and less flow in the periphery, as compared to anger.

Following Darwin's perspective, Ekman (1971, p.216) suggested that "what is universal in facial expressions of emotion is the particular set of facial muscular movements triggered when a given emotion is elicited". Ekman and Friesen (1975) have proposed that, at the morphological level, facial expressions of emotion are best described by changes in one or more areas of the face which can move separately: forehead and eyebrows, eyes and lids, and root of the nose, for the upper face, and cheeks, chin, mouth, nose, for the lower face. These authors have developed a classification of facial muscular movements, the Facial Action Coding System (FACS, Ekman and Friesen, 1978). The FACS is " a comprehensive, anatomically based system for measuring all visually discernible facial movements" (Rosenberg, 1997, p.12). It describes 44 action units (movements of a specific part of the face which can involved several muscles), each of them being also coded in terms of intensity on a 5-point intensity scale. For instance, the main facial movement of the smile, lifting the lip corner toward the ear (through activation of the *Zygomatic Major* muscle) is coded as action unit 12 and the main facial movement of the anger, lowering brow (through activation of *Depressor Glabellae, Depressor Supercilli* and *Corrugator Supercilli*) is coded 4.

Using FACS, Ekman and Friesen (1975) have proposed that specific action unit combinations are associated with emotions. They have described the prototypical displays for seven basic emotions. Evidences of the prototypicality of an action unit combination for a given emotion came from cross-cultural and developmental data (Ekman, 1971; Ekman and Friesen, 1975). Initially, Ekman (1971) observed emotional facial expression of members of two preliterate cultures in New Guinea and concluded that some facial movements were elicited by the same emotion in Western and preliterate cultures, but that others movements were very dissimilar. In that context, Ekman and his colleagues (Ekman, 1971, Ekman and Friesen, 1975) have proposed a neuro-cultural theory of facial expression of emotion (Ekman, 1971). This theory accounts for the observation that basic facial expressions, supposed to be innate, are likely to be modified by experience and socialization and thus vary through cultures. "Display rules", varying from cultures to cultures, (Ekman, 1971, 1973) mediate the link between facial expression and emotional feeling. They can be defined as norms, which "has been learned, presumably fairly early in life, about which management techniques to be applied by whom, to which emotions, under what circumstances". (Ekman, 1971, p.225) They can interfere with the innate affect programs by modifying the expression of emotion: Ones can stop the emotional expression elicited by an event (e.g., poker players do not express any emotion whatever the deal is); ones can exaggerate (e.g. a teacher can fix a troublesome pupil to scold him) or minimize (e.g. a lot of people tend to mask their sadness when they are with others) the felt emotion by intensifying or diminishing features of facial expression; ones can hide an emotion by displaying another emotion (e.g. a person can display a smile when she receives a gift she doesn't like).

Although Ekman's neurocultural model is acknowledged as one of the important theory of emotion, some authors have pointed to the limits of the model. For example, Fridlund (1994) has underlined the over-inclusiveness of the model and the lack of independent criteria to determine in which conditions each component of the model (facial affect program, display rules) is activated. Moreover, Fridlund (1994) has stressed the circularity of Ekman's model. Ekman has developed a rationale in which facial expressions are universal because there are elicited by basic emotion (Ekman, 1971) and he called "basic emotions", emotions that activate a specific facial expression (Ekman, 1992). The concept of display rule is easily used to account for exception in the theoretical perfect matching between primary emotion and emotional facial expression.

Notwithstanding these criticisms, the Facial Action Coding System (Ekman and Friesen, 1975) remains a very valuable tool for the description of emotional facial expressions.

Regarding the focus of this chapter, we will briefly describe the action units involved in anger and fear displays. Examples of prototypical facial displays are shown in Figures 1 and 2. In anger, eyebrows are drawn down and together; this movement produces vertical wrinkles between brows. The lower lids are tensed and may be raised whereas the upper lids are also tensed and may be lowered. The gaze is fixed and seems to be hard. In the upper face, the lips may be either pressed firmly together either the mouth is opened or the lips are tensed in a squarish shape. The nostrils may be dilated. In fear, the eyebrows are raised and drawn together. Horizontal wrinkles cross the centre of forehead. The eyes are largely opened with the eyelid raised and the lower eyelid drawn up. Mouth is the place where the intensity of fear can be observed. The mouth is always opened but either the lips are tensed slightly or stretched and drawn back.

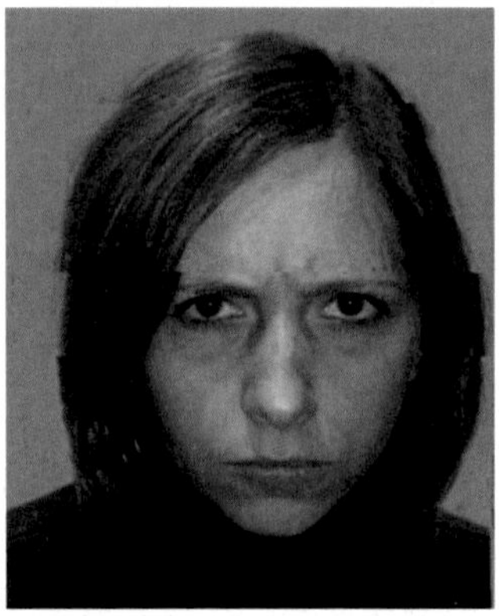

Figure 1. Facial expression of anger

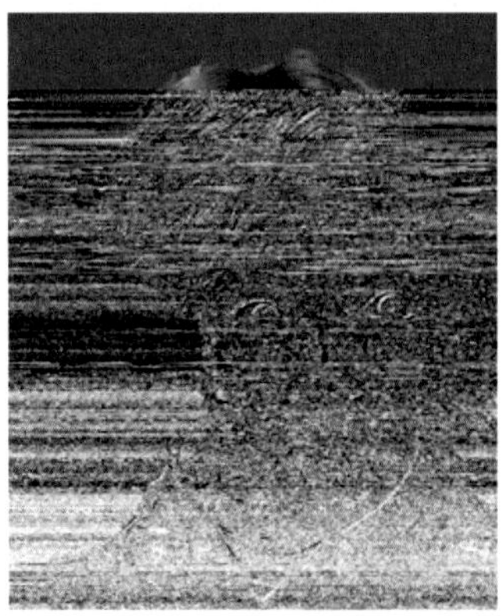

Figure 2. Facial expression of fear

In this section, we have presented a tool, the FACS (Ekman and Friesen, 1975), that describes facial movements involved in the expression of emotion. We also presented Ekman's neurocultural theory accounting for neural, innate and cultural determinants of emotional facial expression and the limits of this model. In the next section, we will focus on the decoding of facial expression. Research on this topic has investigated whether individuals, regardless of their culture, can decode accurately emotional facial expression.

Facial Expression Decoding

Human have an innate ability to process faces, both in terms of identity and expressivity (Russell and Ferández-Dols, 1997). The ability to identify one's emotional state from his or her facial expression develops from birth to adolescence (Gross and Ballif, 1991; Nelson and de Haan, 1997). This assumption comes partly from studies on facial expression decoding. Studies on this topic have been largely initiated by Ekman as well as by Izard and their collaborators.

Researchers have used different types of methodologies to study the decoding of facial expression of emotion. The most used method is the "judgment approach". Subjects are presented with pictures of facial emotional expression and are asked, either to choose a label from a list of emotion words to describe the face ("forced-choice method") or to freely attribute an emotional label to the face ("free-response-method") (Ekman, 1971; Ekman and Friesen, 1975). A common measure for the decoding of emotional facial expressions is defined as the percentage of subjects who attribute to the facial expression the label corresponding to the emotion predicted by the experimenter. One of the limitations of the "forced choice method" (for a critical review, see Fridlund, 1994) is that the categories, provided by the experimenter, rely on the classical distinction of "basic emotions" (Ekman, 1982).

As mentioned above, several researchers (Ekman, 1992; Izard, 1992) contend that facial expressions of emotion have a universal basis. To test this hypothesis, studies, using the methods just described, have been conducting with participants from Western and non Western literate cultures. Taken together, these studies have shown that, regardless of their culture, individuals are able to recognize emotion in facial expression at greater than chance level. However recognition scores vary according to the features of the displayed emotion, the culture, the education level and the measurement method (e.g., facial stimuli sampling, response format).

The best recognized emotion in both Western and non-Western cultures is "happiness" with median scores of correct recognition of respectively 96.4% and 89.2%. (for a review, see Russell, 1994). Curiously, fear has one of the lowest recognition score, 77.5%, in Western culture (65%, in non Western culture) while anger is the worst recognized emotion in non-Western culture with a score of 65% (81.2% in western culture). According to Matsumoto (1992), the difference in recognition rates are not due to absence of universality for emotional expressions but are determined by display rules, i.e., culturally learned rules about how emotions can be expressed and recognized.

Another factor influencing recognition rate is the education level. Wolfgang and Cohen (1988) have shown that the higher the education level, the higher the decoding score with 81 % for people with an university level, 43% for those with only a primary school education.

Finally, Russell (1994, p.235) has concluded from a large literature review that "only the forced choice method supports that, across individuals from (literate) cultures, a very high proportion of subjects agree on a specific emotion for each of hypothesized facial expression". This conclusion is more cautious than Ekman's assumption of universality.

Emotional Responses to Threat Relevant Facial Expressions

In the previous section, we have reviewed studies showing that individuals are able to accurately recognize emotional facial expression in terms of "basic emotions". Research has also documented that individuals react to the facial expressions of their partner, in terms of subjective, physiological, and behavioural responses, as well as in terms of their own facial expression. Such observations are consistent with Seligman's theory of "preparedness" (1971) that states that individuals are prepared to react emotionally to different social situations that are important for the survival of the species, such as face-to-face interaction. In the following sections, we will review the literature relevant to this topic.

Autonomic Responses to Facial Expression

Studies on autonomic conditioning to facial stimuli have documented that some emotional facial expressions possess particular features with respect to evaluative conditioning. In these studies (for a review, see Dimberg, 1988; Öhman, Dimberg and Öst, 1985; Öhman, 1999), subjects were exposed to photographs of facial emotional expressions displaying happy, angry or neutral feeling states. These pictures were used as conditioned stimuli (CSs) associated to an aversive unconditioned stimulus (UCS; electrical shocks on the fingers). Dependant variables were skin conductance responses and heart rate measured during three phases: an habituation phase in which the faces were simply shown to subjects, an acquisition phase in which faces of a specific valence (happy, angry or neutral faces according to the experimental condition) were associated to the aversive stimulus (electrical shock) whereas other faces were not followed by the shock, and finally, an extinction phase in which faces were not followed by a shock. According to the "preparedness" theory (Seligman, 1971), the more a situation is likely to be dangerous, the more individuals are prepared to react rapidly and strongly to it. Given that people expressing anger could represent a potential danger, angry faces should induce more persistent aversive response during the extinction phase compared to happy and neutral face.

In their 1978's study, Öhman and Dimberg observed that the skin conductance responses conditioned to angry faces were more resistant to extinction than those conditioned to happy or neutral faces. In several following studies (Dimberg, 1986; Lanzetta and Orr, 1980, 1981), it was observed that angry faces had an excitatory effect whereas happy face have an inhibitory effect on aversively conditioned responses (Lanzetta and Orr, 1981). Other factors were determinant for the resistant conditioning of angry face: orientation of the head, eye contact and the identity of the person whose face was conditioned(for a review, see Dimberg, 1988; Öhman, Dimberg and Öst, 1985). All these factors are particularly critical in face-to-face interaction. They inform individuals whether they are the target of aggressive threatening intents expressed by the angry face of the interaction partner and thus, whether it is adapted to respond by fear to the anger display.

Facial Reactions to Facial Expression

Studies presented above have focused on the autonomic components of emotional reaction to facial expressions. They supported the hypothesis that human beings are biologically prepared to associate angry face, but not happy face, with aversive consequences. Another component is also particularly relevant to social interaction: the expressive response.

Indeed, in face-to-face interaction, the partners react to each other facial expressions by displaying facial expressions in return (Dimberg, 1997). Mimicry is a concept particularly relevant for this issue. Regarding our specific interest, facial mimicry could be defined as the imitation of an "interaction's partner facial expression" (Hess, Philippot and Blairy, 1999). In this perspective, the question is whether, when exposed to emotional facial expressions, individuals display congruent facial expressions.

This component of emotional reaction had been mostly studied with the technique of electromyography (EMG). This technique allows for the measure of subtle muscle reactions elicited by a broad range of stimuli in different situations. In EMG studies, subjects are repeatedly exposed to different visual or auditory stimuli while surface electrodes record the muscle activity over specific facial regions, such the *Corrugator Supercilii* and *Zygomatic Major* muscle regions. This technique was first developed to measure facial reaction during emotion induction (Lanzetta, Cartwright-Smith, and Kleck, 1976). Cacioppo and Petty (1981) and Schwartz , Fair, Salt, Mandel, and Klemer. (1976) have reported evidences that negative emotions increase the *Corrugator Supercilii* muscle activity whereas positive emotions increase the *Zygomatic Major* muscle activity. Dimberg and co-workers (Dimberg, 1982; Dimberg and Thunberg, 1998; Dimberg, Thumberg and Elmehed, 2000) used EMG to measure facial reaction to the presentation of emotional facial expression. Subjects were exposed to pictures of happy and angry faces. Results have indicated that angry faces increase *Corrugator Supercilii* activity whereas happy faces decrease *Corrugator Supercilii* activity and increase *Zygomatic Major* activity. This pattern is congruent with the result found during emotion induction. This differential muscle activity occurred after only 500 ms of exposure (Dimberg and Thunberg, 1998) and even after a subliminal exposure (Dimberg, Thunberg and Elmhed, 2000). In the latter study, subjects were randomly assigned to 3 different groups according to the valence of the faces displayed (happy-neutral, neutral-neutral or angry-neutral). The exposure of the target face was brief (30 ms) and followed by a neutral masking face displayed during 5 s, in order to prevent any conscious perception of the faces. Results showed that, in the happy-neutral group as compared to angry-neutral group, the activation of *Zygomatic Major* muscle was larger and the activation of *Corrugator Supercilii* muscle was lower.

Taken together, these data suggest that individuals respond with different patterns of facial muscle activity when exposed to different emotional facial expression. In other words, these results confirm that individuals tend to mimic the emotional facial expression they are observing in others.

Behavioral Responses to Facial Expression

Given the importance of threat expression, one could suppose that face processing must enable a rapid detection of potential threatening expression in the environment. Hansen and Hansen (1998) have proposed a research program to test this hypothesis. They used the paradigm of the visual research task developed in experimental psychology for distinguishing between automatic and controlled processing (Shiffrin and Schneider, 1977). They hypothesized that an angry face in a crowd of happy faces should be more easily detected than a happy face in a crowd of angry faces. In this experiment, subjects were presented with an array of 4 or 9 faces. In half of the trials, all the faces had the same emotional expression and in the remaining trials, there was one discrepant face. Subjects were asked to detect the presence of a discrepant face, that is, the face displaying a different emotional expression, in an array of photographs.

Their findings supported the hypothesis of an anger superiority effect: An angry face was more easily detected in a happy or neutral crowd than a happy or neutral face in an angry crowd (Experiments 1 and 3). Moreover, reaction time to detect an angry face in a happy crowd was shorter than the detection time of a happy face in an angry crowd. This asymmetry increased with the size of the crowd. In a similar task (experiment 2), subjects had to identify verbally the location of a discrepant face among a crowd of 4 photographs. The crowd was followed by a mask. The location threshold, that is the necessary exposure duration of the crowd for correct location, was measured. It was found that correct location threshold for an angry face in a happy crowd was lower than the threshold for a happy face in an angry crowd. From these results, despite the evidence of an impact of the size of the crowd, Hansen and Hansen (1988) drew the conclusion that threatening faces pop out of crowds and that this detection is automatic.

Fox and al. (2000) have raised several problems regarding the conclusion drawn by Hansen and Hansen (1988). Firstly, the "face in the crowd" effect doesn't allow to determine whether angry faces are quicker to detect *per se* or whether the effect is determined by the increase of search time through angry distracters. Fox and al. (2000) have underlined methodological problems with material: By controlling contrast artefact (e.g. dark spot on the chin of the angry faces), Purcell, Stewart and Skov (1996) failed to replicate the Hansen and Hansen' s results. Moreover, other studies also failed to replicate the "face in the crowd effect" (Nothdurft, 1993; White, 1995) or have found inconsistent results (Hampton, Purcell, Bersine, Hansen and Hansen, 1989; Suzuki and Cavanagh, 1992). Fox and al. (2000) conducted a series of five experiments designed to test whether angry faces are detected more efficiently. They used the visual search task with schematic faces. They replicated the "face-in-in the crowd effect" with angry schematic faces: angry faces were more easily detected through a matrix of four faces, displaying neutral expression or happiness (Fox and al., 2000; experiments 1, 2, 4 and 5) than the reverse. In contrast to the objection addressed to Hansen and Hansen (1988), these findings cannot be accounted for by low level features of the display: When displays were inverted (faces presented "upside down"), preventing configural processing of emotional expressions, there were no reaction time differences between angry face in neutral crowd and happy face in neutral crowd. (Fox and al., 2001; experiment 3).

Taken together, these results suggest that angry expressions are more efficiently and rapidly detected, compared to happy face. However, the present evidences do not allow to conclude that this detection advantage is automatic in the sense of automaticity developed by Shiffrin and Schneider (1977).Indeed, the fact that detection of angry faces was affected by the crowd size suggested serial rather than parallel processes. More globally, these results support the evolutionary view according to which individuals have the ability to detect efficiently in their environment stimuli relevant for their survival, in this case, angry faces.

Cognitive Formulations of Anxiety

In the previous section, we have reported evidences supporting the assumption that "the key purpose or function of anxiety is probably to facilitate the detection of danger or threat in potentially threatening environments" (Eysenck, 1992, p.4), in order to allow individuals to initiate effective responses to avoid danger. Research has shown that the pre-attentive processing of biologically relevant stimuli, such as photographs of angry faces, orients attentional resources towards threatening stimuli in all individuals. In this section, we will develop the notion that threatening information, including threatening facial expression processing, plays a particularly important role for individuals suffering of emotional disorder.

This assumption, based on an evolutionary perspective, is central to the development of cognitive models of anxiety disorders. There is an evident survival value for the rapid detection of danger cues. Cognitive models of anxiety (e;g; Mogg and Bradley, 1998) postulate that anxious individuals tend to overestimate threat in their environment and to become hypervigilant to threatening signals. Differences in emotional information processing could be a causal factor in the development and the maintenance of emotional disorder (Mathews and Mac Leod, 1994). Before reviewing empirical evidences documenting such biases in the processing of threatening facial expression in anxiety disorders, we will present relevant cognitive and cognitive-motivational models of anxiety.

The first cognitive models of anxiety were developed aside from experimental cognitive psychology and cognitive science. Clinician psychologists (e.g. Beck, Rush, Shaw, and Emery, 1979) concluded from their clinical observations that cognitive processes were impaired in emotional disorders and elaborated a therapy based on the modification of cognitive impairments. This "clinical intuition" has since then been partly supported by a broad range of empirical data relating cognitive factors to emotional disorders (Clark, 1999).

Beck's Schema-Based Model of Anxiety (1976; 1979; 1985)

One of the most popular formulations of emotional disorder had been proposed by Beck (1976). Although the Beckian cognitive approach has received many criticisms (e.g., Teasdale, 1993) that we will present latter, and although Beck (1996) has recently proposed an update of his model, it remains important to present the first version of his model because it is still the most commonly used by therapists.

Beck's first theory of emotional disorders (1976) was quite simple and linear and relied on a definition of the concept of "cognition" coming from common sense, that is consciously experienced images and thoughts. He proposed that (unpleasant) emotions result from (distorted) conscious cognitions. The model is schematically represented in Figure 3.

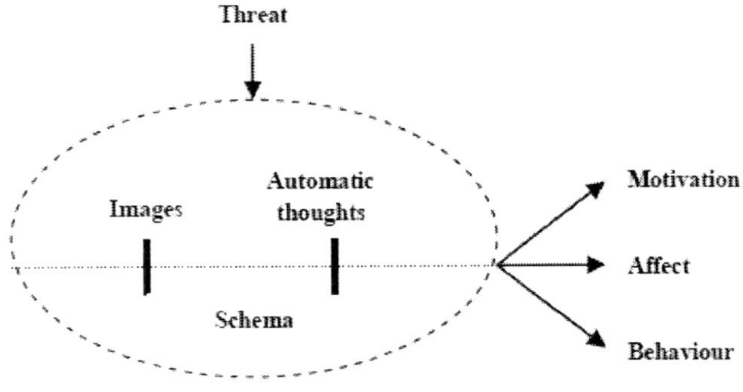

Figure 3. Beck's model (according to Beck, Rush, Shaw, and Emery, 1979)

Specifically for anxious disorders, Beck, Emery, and, Greenberg (1985) proposed that the individuals' response to a threat situation depends on a rapid analysis of the risk of the situation and on their capacity to cope with it. In this perspective, the organism has learned, through previous similar experiences, to recognize a threat situation and the best way to cope with it. This information would be encoded in a schema. The *schema* is a central component of Beck's model. Several definition of the schema can be found in the literature (Bouchard and Freeston, 1995). The definition given by cognitive therapies must be distinguished to the concept of schema developed within cognitive sciences. In the context of cognitive therapies, a schema is a general and stable structure of beliefs that can take a declarative form. In contrast, in multi-level models of emotions (Leventhal, 1984; Teasdale, 1996), the notion of schema refers to an abstract and implicit representation structure, non-declarative in nature (Philippot, Baeyens, Douilliez, and Francart, 2004).

With reference to the former definition of a schema, Beck and al. (1985) suggested that emotional disorders are determined by dysfunctional schemas. For instance, in social anxiety, individuals would hold dysfunctional beliefs, emanating from their schema, about themselves and how they must behave in social situation (e.g., "If I show that I feel anxious, I will look ridiculous", "if I am not perfect, other will not love me" or "I am useless"). When activated by a stressful event, for example a public speech situation, the content of the schema would influence individuals' perception, interpretation and memory towards schema-congruent information and organize emotional, motivational and behavioural responses. Anxiety prone individuals would be biased towards threat in the selection and processing of schema-congruent stimuli (we will review evidences of such biases in the next section). For instance, socially anxious individuals would perceive more quickly that a conversation partner is frowning than would non-anxious individuals. This selective bias is accompanied of a set of physiological responses. According to Beck and al. (1985), dysfunctional schemas are maintained by judgment errors, such as the overestimation of probability ("If I give a speech, I will stutter"), the overestimation of negative outcomes ("If I blush, everybody makes fun of me") or dichotomous though ("If my speech is not perfect, I am stupid). Moreover, by focusing only on schema-congruent information, anxious individuals sustain the schema activation and are unable to detect information disconfirming their erroneous beliefs (e.g., anxious individuals don't realize that a lot of people are in fact interested in their speech).

Undoubtedly, the Beck's model has offered an interesting framework for earlier efficient treatments of anxiety and depression but it also raises several of problems. We summarize here Teasdale's criticisms (1993): (a) Negative thinking is not an antecedent of depression, as postulated by Beck, but a consequence of it. This claim is suggested by the fact that research has shown that anti-depressant drugs as well as other efficient treatments of depression--that are not targeting negative thinking--are as efficient as cognitive therapy in reducing negative thinking. (b) Irrational believes, assumed to be a specific predisposing factor for emotional disorder, can be activated by inducing a corresponding mood state in healthy individuals. Therefore, schema activation is mood-dependent rather than an enduring feature of vulnerability. (c) Although Beck postulates a necessary mediating links between though and emotion, people can feel an emotion without being able to identify the related negative though. (d) Most patients "rationally" know that their believes are irrational (e.g. "Rationally, I know that nobody will reject me if I am blushing… ") and, consequently, giving rational arguments as advocated by Beck is not efficient to change "emotional" believes (e.g. "…but emotionally. I feared to be rejected"). Moreover, the schema-based model doesn't account for difference in processing biases found between anxiety and depression (Mogg and Bradley, 1998). Indeed, there are empirical evidences for attentional biases in anxiety disorders. Anxious individuals preferentially process negative information (for a review, see Mogg and Bradley, 1998), and for memory biases in depression: Depressed patients have a recall advantage for negative material (Mac Leod, 1990), whereas research has failed to find consistent memory biases in anxiety (Mac Leod, 1999) or attentional biases in depression (Wells and Mathews, 1994)

Other problems can be mentioned. For instance, Beck's definition of cognition as "any ideation with verbal or pictorial content" (Beck, 1979) that might be conscious does not account for implicit cognition. Moreover, Philippot (2000) has also criticized the notion of continuum between preconscious and conscious thoughts assuming that cognitive processes are similar in nature. Indeed, these processes could be from a different nature.

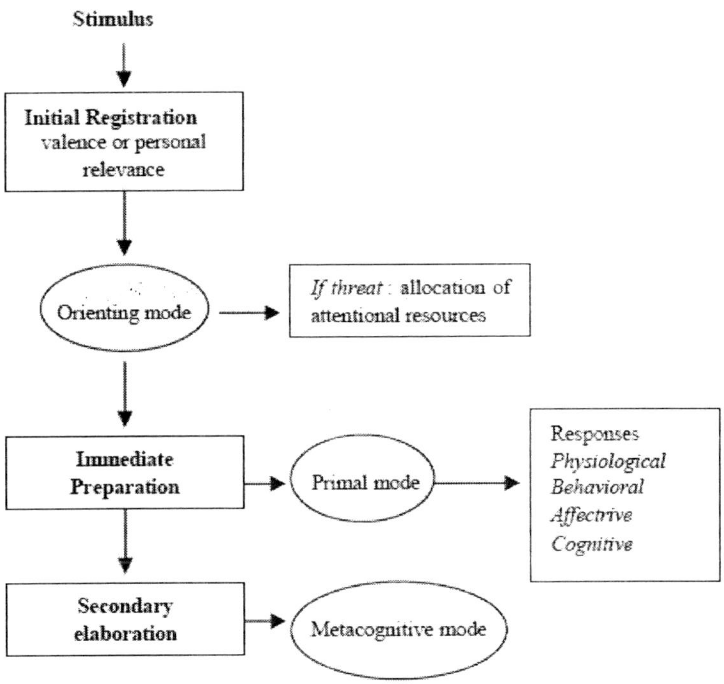

Figure 4. The three-stage schema–based information processing model of anxiety (Beck and Clark, 1997)

In a recent reformulation of his model, Beck and Clark (1997) have proposed a three-stage schema-based information model of anxiety that attempts to address previous criticisms. These different stages imply different levels of automaticity from rapid, involuntary, and unconscious processes to controlled, strategic, and elaborative processes (for a definition of automaticity related to anxious disorders, see Mc Nally, 1995). The model is schematically represented in Figure 4. The first processing stage, *initial registration,* involved an automatic recognition of the valence or the personal relevance of stimuli, named *orienting mode.* If the stimulus is assessed as threatening, attentional resources are allocated to process it. In anxiety, the orienting mode is hypersensitive to detect negative stimuli. For example, when giving a speech, a socially anxious individual would appraise negatively the yawns of an audience 's member. This appraisal activates an orienting mode of danger. The attentional resources are oriented towards this threatening stimulus. Empirical evidences support the notion of a bias towards negative stimuli in preattentive processing in anxiety (for a review, see Mogg and Bradley, 1998).

The second stage, *immediate preparation*, involves the activation of a *primal mode* that triggers a series of physiological, behavioural, affective and cognitive responses. In anxiety, this primal mode results in biased cognitive processing, such as hypervigilance to threat cues rather than safety cues and automatic negative thoughts.

Finally, the *secondary elaboration* stage is characterized by a full semantic activation as well as the activation of other relevant schema. Individuals activate a metacognitive mode in which they evaluate the availability and the efficiency of their coping resources. This mode of processing is necessarily conscious and explicit.

Beck's conception of anxiety bares important implications for treatment. According to Beck and Clark (1997, p.55), "because (...) threat assignment is the *sine qua non* of anxiety disorders, effective treatments must modify the threat appraisal process". Many clinicians shared the belief that anxious individuals overestimate the threat meaning of trivial stimuli and aim to modify such erroneous "decoding" using verbally mediated therapy, like cognitive therapies. However, Mc Nally (1995) raised doubt on the capacity of cognitive therapies, based on conscious verbally processes to modify cognitive biases that are automatic. By contrast, Mansell (2000) reviewed evidences for a modification of automatic processes by conscious appraisal.

Mogg and Bradley's Cognitive-Motivational Model (1998)

In order to account for differences in cognitive biases in depression versus anxiety, as postulated by Beck and al. (1985), Mogg and Bradley (1998) have proposed to examine two factors largely developed in psychobiological and personality theories: the emotional valence and the goal engagement. Within this two-dimensional framework, depression is characterized by a negative valence of the environment (e.g., lack of pleasure and interest) and a disengagement from external goals with a cognitive focus on the internal life (e.g., towards depressive thoughts). Anxiety is also characterized by a negative valence of the environment (e.g., threatening and likely dangerous) but is conversely characterized by an engagement towards external goals (e.g., preparation to escape from the aversive situation)

According to the distinction between these two factors, Mogg and Bradley (1998) have proposed a cognitive-motivational view of anxiety. They distinguished two motivational systems that mediate cognitive and behavioural responses to emotional stimuli: the Valence Evaluation System and the Goal Engagement System. The Valence Evaluation System automatically assesses the stimulus threat value according to the nature of the stimulus, the situational context, the person's state anxiety, and prior learning experiences. The Goal Engagement System orients allocation of attention as a function of the output of the former system. If a stimulus in the environment is evaluated as threatening, the Goal Engagement System interrupts ongoing activities and orients attention toward the threat stimulus. This model thus postulates that attentional biases in anxious individuals result from a negative and automatic appraisal of social situations (Mogg and Bradley, 2002).

This cognitive-motivational view of anxiety is quite similar to the model proposed by Williams, Watts, MacLeod, and Mathews (1988). This latter model is also based on two mechanisms, the Affective Decision Mechanism and the Resource Allocation Mechanism. These two mechanisms have similar functions as Mogg and Bradley' s systems presented above. The only important difference between these models rests in the system that determine vulnerability to anxiety. According to Williams and al. (1988), individual differences in vulnerability to anxiety (anxiety trait) influence the Resource Allocation Mechanism. Thus, high trait anxious individuals have a tendency to orient their attention towards threat, whereas low trait anxious individuals shift their attention away from threat. According to Mogg and Bradley's model, individual differences in vulnerability to anxiety would be due to a greater sensitivity of the Valence Evaluation System. Thus, anxiety-prone individuals would tend to over-estimate the threat value of stimuli that would be assessed as trivial by low anxious individuals.

In summary, the cognitive-motivational view (Mogg and Bradley, 1998) postulates that attentional biases in anxious individuals result from a negative and automatic appraisal of situations (Mogg and Bradley, 2002). Anxious individuals would appraise their anxiogenic stimuli as more negative and would consequently allocate more attention to them than non anxious individuals would.

Empirical Evidence of Fearful Processing Biases in Anxiety

The models of anxiety disorders described in the previous section are based on empirical evidences coming from studies using paradigms of experimental cognitive psychology. Several studies were conducted on general cognitive deficits in the processing of complex information, regardless of its emotional valence in anxiety. However, in this chapter, we will specifically focus on studies concerning the processing of emotional, and particularly fear-relevant, information. These studies have evidenced processing biases for threatening information in clinical and sub-clinical anxious samples. These cognitive biases appear to affect all processing levels: attention, memory, and interpretation.

We will now reviewed studies relevant for the purpose of this chapter, that is studies focused on fearful facial expression in anxiety disorders. Some of these studies have focused on a particular anxious disorder, social phobia. Indeed, there is a strong belief that faces are specifically relevant for social phobics. Actually, the basic fear in social phobia is about being negatively evaluated by others. Facial expression constitutes a central medium for conveying positive and negative evaluations in face-to-face interactions. Thus, they are particularly relevant for social phobics.

Attentional Biases

Studies focusing on attentional processes have mainly used three types of paradigms: the emotional Stroop task, the probe detection task and the face-in-the crowd task. In most of these studies, words were used as material, but some studies, using the probe detection task or the face in the crowd task, used faces as stimuli.

The Probe Detection Task

The paradigm of probe detection was proposed by Mac Leod, Mathews and Tata (1986) in order to offer a more direct measurement of the allocation of the visual attention than in the Stroop task. The probe detection task is based on a paradigm coming from the cognitive psychology according to which the spatial attention can be evaluated through reaction time to visual signals (Navon and Margalit, 1983; Posner, Snyder and Davidson, 1980), i.e. individuals tend to respond faster to a signal presented in the attended area of the visual field. Typically, pairs of stimuli are presented on a screen, one below the other or one beside the other. In critical trials, a stimulus is emotional and the other neutral. Each pair is presented during a fixed time (generally 500 ms). When the pair disappears, a probe stimulus (a dot or an arrow pointing either up or down) appears in the area previously occupied by one of the two stimuli. The subject is asked to press as quickly and accurately as possible one of two keys corresponding to the location of the dot or to the direction of the arrow. Shorter reaction time when the probe is located on the area previously occupied by a given stimulus reveals an attentional bias towards this type of stimulus.

This paradigm has allowed to evidence the presence of attentional bias towards threatening words in generalized anxious disorder (Mac Leod, Mathews and Tata, 1986, Mogg, Mathews and Eysenck, 1992) and social phobia (Asmundson and Stein, 1994). A similar bias was also reported in non pathological anxiety (Mogg, Bradley, de Bono and Painter, 1997; Mac Leod and Mathews, 1988).

Notwithstanding this robust evidence, several researchers (Mogg and Bradley, 1999) have underlined the lack of ecological validity of words and have proposed the use of emotional faces as stimuli. The latter are particularly ecological and relevant stimuli for any human being (Mogg and Bradley, 1998). As developed in previous sections, individuals have a particular and innate capacity to process human faces (Dimberg, 1988; Öhman, Dimberg and Öst, 1985).

We have reviewed twelve studies using the probe detection task with faces to test the hypothesis of an attentional bias for threatening information in clinical and non clinical samples. When the stimulus duration is 500 ms, high trait anxious individuals show a vigilance bias for angry faces (Bradley, Mogg, Falla and Hamilton, 1998; Mogg and Bradley, 1999; Mogg, Philippot and Bradley, 2004) and for fear faces (Fox, 2002, experiment 1). Similar results are observed for longer exposure durations (1100 ms or 1250 ms) for high trait anxious individuals (Bradley and al., 1998) and for high-state anxious individuals (Bradley, Mogg and Millar, 2000).

Presentations of masked faces in the probe detection task were used to test whether anxiety-related biases might imply processes outside awareness. Mogg and Bradley (1999, experiment 3, 2002) and Fox (2002) reported that high-trait anxious individuals have an increased tendency to orient attention towards the spatial location of negative faces displayed under subliminal conditions.

These findings were replicated among patients suffering from generalized anxiety (Bradley, Mogg, White, Groom, and de Bono, 1999) regardless the stimuli duration (500 or 1250 ms). The generalized anxious patients selectively attended to threatening facial expressions, but they were also more vigilant than controls for emotional faces in general. This study also showed a complex pattern of attentional bias towards the happy faces. The social anxiety scores of the participants were positively correlated with attentional bias scores for threat in all tasks.

The previous findings underline the crucial role of processing threatening facial expressions in social anxiety. Bradley Mogg, and Millar (2000) reported that high levels of social anxiety predict an attentional bias for threatening faces. This study assessed the orienting of initial eye movement during a probe detection task. This measure was recorded by using eye tracker sensors positioned below the right eye. However, Bradley, Mogg, Millar, Bonham-Carter, Fergusson, Jenkins, and Parr (1997) did not find attentional bias for angry faces when the students were divided in two groups on the basis of social anxiety measures. Mansell, Clark, Ehler and Chen (1999) have found a significant an attentional bias but in the opposite direction: Socially anxious individuals showed an attentional bias away from emotional faces (not only threatening faces). The task used was slightly different from the one used in previous experiments. One difference rests in the material presented. In the "classical" probe detection task, participants were presented with neutral-happy and neutral-angry face pairs. In contrast, in Mansell's study, the negative (anger, dislike, fear, sadness), happy or neutral faces were paired with a photograph of neutral household object. The second difference is that participants were assigned either to a social-evaluative threat condition, that is, a condition within they believed they would give a speech, or to a no-threat condition. Under condition of social-evaluative threat, high socially anxious individuals showed an attentional bias away from emotional faces whereas under the no threat condition, high and low socially anxious individuals did not differ from each other. However, in the no threat condition, attentional bias scores were positively correlated with trait anxiety. High-trait anxiety individuals showed an enhanced vigilance bias to negative faces. This latter result is consistent with studies previously described (Bradley, Mogg and Millar, 2000; Fox, 2002; Mogg and Bradley, 1999; Mogg, Philippot and Bradley, 2004). These results suggest that socially anxious individuals, under condition of social-evaluative threat situation, avoid positive and negative faces more than neutral ones. As Bradley et al. (1999) as well as Mansell et al. (1999) suggested that socially anxious individuals react in the same way to happy and negative faces because both can be seen as potentially threatening. But the direction of the postulated bias is different. In contrast to Bradley et al. (1999), Mansell et al. (1999) suggest that socially anxious individuals shift their attention away from emotional faces and increase their self-focused-attention. This pattern could enhance anxiety, generate negative images of themselves and contribute to the maintenance of social anxiety (Clark and Wells, 1995).

The studies presented just above were conducted in sub-clinical samples, that is individuals high in the social-anxiety-trait but without reaching the criterion defined in the DSM IV (APA, 1994). Studies conducted on clinical samples might help in resolving the contradictions observed in the results of sub-clinical studies, i.e. whether the attention is oriented towards or away from threatening faces in social phobics. Chen, Ehlers, Clark and Mansell (2002) have presented faces and household objects simultaneously for 500 ms to 20 social phobics and 20 normal controls. They have found that social phobics directed their attention away from the faces, regardless of emotional expression and towards household objects. Mogg, Philippot and Bradley (2004) found the reverse pattern of results. Social phobics and matched controls completed a probe detection task with only facial expressions as stimuli and no household objects. Moreover, in order to observe whether or not the focus of attention changed over time, the stimulus duration was manipulated (either 500 ms or 1250 ms). Results indicated that, in the 500ms condition, the same duration as in the Chen's et al. (2002) study, social phobics showed an initial attentional bias towards angry faces, relative to happy and neutral faces. In the 1250 ms condition, this bias disappeared. It is important to stress the difference in control stimuli (neutral face vs household object) in those two studies as well as between the Mansell and al. (1999) and Bradley and al (1997)' s studies. A possible explanation for these discrepant results is that, when socially anxious individuals have inanimate objects in their environment, they attend to those non social stimuli rather than to faces.

In order to reconciliate these different findings, Amir, Freshman, and Foa (2002) have proposed a two-stage model of information processing. According to this view, anxious individuals would show an initial hypervigilance focus for threat-relevant stimuli. This hypervigilance would be the consequence of automatic processes and it could be observed without conscious perception of threat relevant information (Mogg and Bradley, 1999). However, at further and less automatic stages of information processing, people would actively turn away from threatening information to escape the discomfort associated with it. This model thus postulates a dynamic shift of attention allocation from initial threat hypervigilance to later threat avoidance. For instance, while speaking to other people, socially anxious individuals would have their attention automatically attracted to frown more readily than non anxious individuals. Because of this perception bias, socially anxious individuals are likely to automatically over-activate a state of social anxiety. However, as soon as a frown would be detected, they would turn away their attention from it, and more generally from others' faces, to avoid the threatening stimulus and the discomfort associated with it. Unfortunately, in doing so, they are likely to maintain their anxiety: Not only are they likely to socially behave inappropriately, but they will also be unable to determine whether the frowns were a sign of actual social threat, or rather just a sign of perplexity, for instance.

In sum, studies using dot probe paradigm showed vigilance towards threatening faces, in generalized anxiety disorder and in sub clinical anxiety measured by the STAI (State-Trait Anxiety Inventory, Spielberger, 1983). The data for clinical and sub-clinical *socially* anxious individuals are less clear. It seems that, when confronted to facial expression material only, socially anxious tend to focus on threatening faces. However, if they have the choice between attending to facial expressions or to non-social object, they attend to non-social object.

The principal limitation of the dot probe task is that it presents a "snapshot" of the attentional bias, depending on stimuli duration. This technique measures the initial orienting of attention but cannot detect attention shifts during stimulus display. Indeed, subjects might repeatedly shift their attention towards and away from threat during exposure to facial expressions (Mogg and Bradley, 1998).

Face in the Crowd. In a previous section, we presented a paradigm, named the "Face in the Crowd" paradigm (Hansen and Hansen, 1988). It was designed to test the assumption that human beings are able to detect efficiently angry faces in their environment. The existence of this "face-in-the-crowd" effect was reported for normal subjects with photographs of emotional faces (Hansen and Hansen, 1988) and with schematic facial expressions (Fox and al., 2000). The evolutionary view of anxiety (Eysenck, 1992) predicts an enhanced ability to detect threat in anxiety.

Byrne and Eysenck (1995) used this paradigm to investigate whether anxious individuals detect more quickly threat than normal controls or not. Their data have established that high-trait anxious individuals were faster than low-trait anxious individuals to detect angry faces in a neutral crowd, whereas the two groups did not differ in detection speed of a happy face in a neutral crowd. Similar results were found in a clinical sample of social phobics (Gilboa-

Schechtman, Foa and Amir, 1999): Compared to controls, social phobics reported a greater attentional bias for angry than for happy faces in a neutral crowd. Moreover, social phobics were slower than controls when making decisions for angry and happy than for neutral crowds. Esteves (1999) has replicated the "anger superiority" effect with schematic facial expressions. However, individuals with high social anxiety measured by the FNE (Fear of Negative Evaluation, Watson and Friend, 1969) and the SADS (Social Avoidance Scale and Distress, Watson and Friend, 1969) failed to display faster detection of angry faces but made more errors than the low anxiety group.

In summary, these studies underline two important aspects of the processing of threatening facial expressions. Firstly, threatening facial expression seem to be better detected in all human beings and to be a particularly fear-relevant stimuli. Secondly, social phobics show a greater detection bias for angry faces. This bias, however, is not shown by sub-clinically socially anxious individuals.

Conclusions

In this section, we have presented evidences coming from several paradigms that generalized anxious individuals and individuals with a high anxiety-trait show an attentional bias towards anger and fear faces. Such evidences support the postulate of cognitive models of anxiety (Beck and al., 1985; Beck and Clark, 1997, Mogg and Bradley, 1998) and are congruent with the evolutionary view (Eysenck, 1992). These results have important implication for the understanding of the factors that maintain anxiety disorders. Indeed, anxious individual, selectively attending to threat information, subjectively perceives the world as more threatening and unsafe than it is. This attentional bias prevents them to attend to other elements in their environment than threat. As a consequence, such aversive perception of the environment reinforces their anxiety. The few data addressing this issue in social phobia didn't resolve the question of the orienting—towards or away—of the attentional bias. More research is needed to specify the role of attentional biases for face - a particularly relevant stimulus- in social phobia.

Evaluative Deficit and Biases in Facial Decoding

In the previous section, we reviewed empirical evidences addressing whether anxious individuals display an attentional bias towards threatening facial expressions. In this section, we will examine whether anxious individuals present an evaluative bias in judging facial expressions. This is, do they over-attribute threat to facial signals? Regarding verbal material, a wealth of research has now shown an interpretative bias toward threatening interpretation of ambiguous stimuli (Mac Leod, 1999). This evidence supports models of anxiety such as those of Beck (1985). Further, Mogg and Bradley's model of anxiety (1998) hypothesizes that attentional biases result from evaluative biases. This notion is widely accepted by clinicians (e.g. Beck, Emery and Greenberg, 1985) but, curiously, has been submitted to very little empirical investigation for nonverbal material. We will demonstrate that the empirical evidences reported by studies conducting on this topic are inconsistent with this hypothesis.

Few studies have been published on evaluative biases in the decoding of emotional facial expression by socially anxious individuals. All these studies used different paradigms. Firstly, Merckelbach, Van Hout, van den Hout, and Mersch (1989) observed no differences between nine social phobics and nine controls in their evaluation of angry, neutral, and joyful faces with respect to pleasantness. Moreover, they didn't observe differences between social phobics and normal controls in psychophysiological reactions (skin conductance response, eyeblink rate) to the presentation of facial stimuli.

Douilliez and Philippot (2003) replicated these results with individuals with a high level of social anxiety as measured by the FNE (Fear of Negative Evaluation, Watson and Friend, 1969): Participants were asked to evaluate the threatening value of angry, joyful, and neutral faces. No differences between anxious individuals and controls were observed for the evaluation of faces.

Using a different procedure, Winton, Clark, and Edelmann (1995) found some differences between socially anxious and non-anxious individuals. Socially anxious and non-anxious students were very briefly (60 ms.) exposed to negative and neutral facial expressions. Following this subliminal presentation, participants had to rate the emotion of each facial expression on a nine-point scale ranging from "negative" to "positive". It appeared that students with high scores of social anxiety detected more accurately negative facial expressions than did non-anxious students while the opposite pattern was observed for neutral expressions. However, further analyses demonstrated that these effects were due to an overall negativity bias in the anxious students, and the authors concluded to an "absence of an enhanced ability to discriminate between different emotional states in others" (p. 193) in their socially anxious participants.

Finally, Philippot and Douilliez (2005) investigated this question with a facial expression decoding task. Participants-- patients with social phobia, patients suffering from anxiety disorders without social phobia and normal controls-- were presented with 40 facial expressions of happiness, anger, sadness, disgust and fear differing in emotional intensity by 30 % steps from neutral to full-blown emotional expression. Participants had to judge each expression on seven-point scales for seven emotions: happiness, anger, sadness, disgust, fear, surprise and shame. No differences between groups were found in the way participants judged emotional facial expressions.

The previous studies were conducting among adults, but some studies have also attempted to relate EFE decoding skills and social anxiety in children. In a sample of 8- to 10-year olds, McClure and Nowicki (2001) did not find a relationship between self-reported social anxiety and the ability to correctly label emotional facial expressions presented for 1 s. In a study similar to Winton et al.'s (1995), Melfsen and Florin (2002) exposed 8- to 12-year olds to emotional facial expressions for 60 ms. These children were asked to guess whether the emotional facial expression presented was positive, neutral, or negative. Compared to non-anxious children, socially anxious children more often reported that they saw emotion when a neutral face was presented. However, there was no indication of an enhanced ability to decode negative facial expressions in socially anxious children, nor was there a specific tendency to interpret neutral or positive faces as negative.

In the previous section, we presented several empirical studies suggesting that socially anxious and phobics individuals are more sensitive to threatening facial expression and would automatically detect more readily such information. According to Mogg and Bradley (1998)'s model, these attentional biases in anxious individuals result from a negative and automatic appraisal of social situations (Mogg and Bradley, 2002).

The results presented here suggested that socially anxious individuals do not process emotional facial expression more thoroughly and that they do not explicitly attribute a different meaning to emotional facial expressions as compared to non-anxious individuals. The present evidences suggest that socially anxious individuals know as well as non anxious that an angry face means anger and a sad face means sadness, for instance. We have proposed (Philippot and Douillez, 2005) that the higher sensitivity in the automatic evaluation of emotional facial expressions in socially anxious individuals would not concern valence per se (this stimulus is more or less negative), but rather personal concern (this stimulus signals something potentially important for the way one might be evaluated by others). This proposition is actually congruent with the model of Mogg and Bradley (1998) who proposed that Valence Evaluation System "integrates information from nonconscious automatic appraisal processes with other information resulting from more detailed, elaborate analyses of stimulus and its context and consequences" (p. 841). The terms " valence evaluation" are thus a bit misleading here, as this system refers to relevance for the person's concerns.

Memory Biases

Very little research as been conducted on memory bias in fear and anxiety. Three studies have used paradigms that involve incidental memory to examine memory biases for threatening EFE. These studies have provided inconclusive results. Lundh and Öst (1996) have observed a recognition bias for "critical" faces by social phobics. Participants--social phobics or normal controls--were initially presented with 20 photographs and were asked to judge whether the person in the photograph was a critical or accepting person (encoding task). Following a distracting task, participants were instructed to look through a file with 80 faces and to identify the 20 persons they had seen in the first task. Social phobics, compared to controls, recognized a higher proportion of critical as compared to accepting face. It is interesting to note that, on the average, social phobics did not rate the faces as more critical than the controls did.

Similarly, Foa, Gilboa-Schechtman, Amir, and Freshman (2000) have observed that socially anxious individuals exhibit a negative memory bias towards threatening emotional facial expression. In experiment 1, participants (generalized social phobics or normal controls) were presented 12 photographs of persons displaying various emotional expressions. In the learning task, they learned the name of the person in the photograph. In a second task of emotional encoding, participants were presented 12 photographs of the same person but displaying another emotional expression than in the first task. They were instructed to name the person and to identify his or her emotional expression. In a free recall task, participants were asked to write down the name of the 12 persons with their emotional expression displayed in the previous task. In the last task, a cued recall task, participants received a list of the names of the 12 persons presented previously and were asked to write down the emotional expression displaying by each person in the second task. Results showed that social phobics, compared to normal controls, exhibit better free recall and cued recalls for facial expression associated with names (cued recall). Socials phobics remembered angry expressions better than did normal controls but there were no significant difference for happy and neutral expressions. In experiment 2, participants were asked, in the learning task, to pay attention for 5 seconds to 12 photographs of person displaying various emotional expressions. In the recognition task, participants were presented the 12 photographs seen in the first task but displaying another emotional expression and 12 photographs of another persons and were instructed to identify "old" (seen in the first task) and "new" photographs. Foa et al. (2000) observed that social phobics, as compared to normal controls, showed a better recognition of facial expressions. Moreover, social phobics presented a recognition bias towards negative emotional expressions. In sum, social phobics exhibited a better recall and recognition for all facial expression, with an enhanced recognition for negative expressions as compared to non-negative expressions.

Perez-Lopez and Woody (2001) failed to observe such a memory bias. Before the encoding task, participants (social phobics or normal controls) were instructed to give a speech in front of a live audience and a video camera. In the encoding task, they were asked to look through a series of photographs of faces displaying threatening and reassurance expressions. After that, participants prepared their speech. In the recognition task, participants were shown two photographs of the same person (a reassuring one and a threatening one) and were asked to indicate which photographs had been previously presented. Socials phobics, compared to normal controls, were less accurate in identifying the expression associated with faces that they had previously seen. This accuracy bias was mediated by the anxiety state generated by the speech task. But, contrary to the results of Lundh and Öst (1996) and Foa, Gilboa-Schechtman, Amir, and Freshman (2000), social phobics did not exhibit a memory bias towards threatening facial expressions.

In this section, we reviewed three studies on memory bias in social phobia using three different methodologies. The results are inconsistent. Fox and al. (2000) and Lundh and Öst (1996) evidenced an enhanced memory for negative faces whereas Pérez-López and Woody (2001) did not observed this bias but showed that social phobics were less accurate than non-anxious controls in a facial recognition memory task.

CONCLUSION

In this chapter, we have presented several lines of research investigating emotional facial expression in normal individuals and in those suffering from anxiety. Studies on decoding and detection of emotional facial expression as well as studies on physiological and expressive responses to emotional facial expression confirmed that human beings have an innate ability to process emotional facial expression, in general, and threatening expression in particular. This conclusion is consistent with the Darwin's evolutionary view of emotion and with Seligman's theory of "preparedness" (1971) that states that individuals are prepared to react emotionally to fear-relevant situation.

At a psychopathological level, many cognitive models postulate that cognitive biases, including evaluative, attentional and memory biases, play a key role in anxiety disorders. Specifically, most cognitive models of anxiety assume that anxious individuals overestimate threat in facial expressions, preferentially allocate attention to threatening face and better recall and recognize negative faces. Some models (e.g. Mogg and Bradley, 1998) postulate a causal link between evaluative and attentional biases: Attentional biases in anxious individuals may result from a negative and automatic appraisal of anxiogenic situations.

While there are strong evidences that generalized anxious individuals and individuals with a high anxiety-trait show an attentional bias towards anger and fear faces, the direction of the bias is less clear for social phobia. Further research is needed to explore the direction of this bias. This issue is particularly important for the comprehension of the most prevalent anxiety disorders: social phobia. In fact, opposed results regarding this bias in social phobia can be found in the literature: some studies evidencing a bias *towards* threatening faces (hypervigilance for threat), others reporting a bias *away* from threatening faces (avoidance). We have shown that these diverging results come from two paradigms differing in their control condition. In the Bradley, Mogg and co-workers's studies, both threatening and control material were facial expressions while in Clark, Chen and co-workers' studies, target stimuli were emotional facial expression and control stimuli household objects. A vigilance bias for threatening facial expression is congruent with several cognitive models of general anxiety (Beck and al., 1985; Mogg and Bradley, 1998) and social phobia (Rapee and Heimberg, 1997) whereas an avoidance bias supports Clark and Wells' (1995) model of social phobia. The latter model suggestes that social phobics avoid external threat cues and focus their attention on internal threat cues (anxiety symptoms). A hypervigilance-avoidance model has been proposed to reconciliate theses discrepant findings (Amir and al., 2002).

Quite evidently, further research has to specify the nature of these attentional biases in social phobia. Firstly, studies should compare allocation of attention to facial expression at different stages of the information processing, in order to determine whether attention allocation shifts from threatening to non-threatening stimuli. Secondly, studies should design, in the same experiment, two control conditions, one with neutral faces, and one with non-facial neutral information. Finally, studies should investigate the competition in attention allocation between external and internal cues.

In any case, several cognitive models (Beck and al., 1985; Mogg and Bradley, 1998) postulate that attentional biases are the consequence of an evaluative bias. In social phobia, Clark and Well's model (1995) suggests a more elaborate bias in the appraisal of social situations: Social phobics would appraise social situations as more threatening because they hold negative assumptions on their ability to behave adequately and on negative consequences of their behaviours. There is also a strong belief among clinicians in the existence of bias or of deficit in the interpretation of others' emotional signals, especially of others' facial expression.

However, despite a clinical belief and theoretical claims, studies we reviewed didn't show an explicit evaluative bias for facial expression in social phobics. This discrepancy between theoretical and clinician believes, on one hand, and experimental evidences, on the other hand, open a debate that is particularly important for treatment perspectives. Should anxious individuals be trained to reappraise more positively anxiogenic situation—a proposal implying that they are biased in their evaluation of such situation? Or, rather, should they be trained to confront and sustain voluntary their attention on threat cues—a proposal implying that their attentional bias plays a major role in the elicitation and maintenance of anxiety? Present evidences seem to favour the latter solution. However, moreresearch is needed to disentangled this Gordian node of anxiety.

AUTHORS' NOTES

The writing of this chapter has been facilitated by grants from the "Fonds National de la Recherche Scientifique de Belgique" 8.4512.98 and 3.4609.01.

The authors appreciate the helpful comments of Raymond Bruyer on earlier drafts of this paper. Correspondence regarding this chapter should be addressed to Electronic mail may be sent via Internet to "Celine.Douilliez@psp.ucl.ac.be" or to "Pierre.Philippot@psp.ucl.ac.be". Recent updates of our research can be found on Internet: www.ecsa.ucl.ac.be/personnel/douilliez/ or on www.ecsa.ucl.ac.be/personnel/philippot/.

REFERENCES

American Psychiatric Association. (1994). *Diagnostic and statistical manual of mental disorders.* (4th ed.). Washington, DC: Author.

Amir, N., Freshman, M. and Foa, E. (2002). Enhanced Stroop interference for threat in social phobia. *Journal of Anxiety disorder, 16*, 1-9.

Asmundson, G.J.G. and Stein, M.B. (1994). Selective processing of social threat in patients with generalized social phobia: Evaluation using a dot-probe paradigm. *Journal of Anxiety Disorders, 8*, 107-117.

Beck, A.T. (1976). *Cognitive therapy and the emotional disorders.* New York: International Universities Press.

Beck, A.T. (1996). Beyond belief: A theory of modes, personality and psychopathology. In P.M. Salkovskis (Ed.), *Frontiers of cognitive therapy* (pp.1-25). New York: Guilford Press.

Beck, A.T. and Clark, D.A. (1997). An information processing model of anxiety: automatic and strategic processes. *Behaviour Research and Therapy,35*, 49-58.

Beck, A.T., Emery, G. and Greenberg, R.L. (1985). Cognitive structures and anxiogenic rules. In A.T., Beck, G., Emery and R.L. Greenberg (Eds), *Anxiety disorders and phobias* (pp. 54-66). New York: Basic books.

Beck, A.T., Rush, A.J., Shaw, B.F. and Emery, G. (1979). *Cognitive therapy of depression: A treatment manual.* New York: Guilford Press.

Bouchard, S. and Freeston, M. (1995). Schéma cognitif et anxiété: I: considérations théoriques et cliniques. *Thérapie Comportementale et Cognitive, 5*, 7-16.

Bradley, B., Mogg, K., Falla, S. and Hamilton, L.(1998). Attentional Bias for Threatening Facial Expressions in Anxiety: Manipulation of Stimulus Duration. *Cognition and Emotion,12* ,737-753.

Bradley, B., Mogg, K., White, J., Groom, C. and de Bono, J. (1999). Attentional bias for emotional faces in generalized anxiety disorder, *British Journal of Clinical Psychology, 38*, 267-278.

Bradley, B.P., Mogg, K., and Millar, N. (2000). Covert and overt orienting of attention to emotional faces in anxiety. *Cognition and Emotion, 14,* 789-808.

Bradley, B.P., Mogg, K., Millar, N.H, Bonham-Carter, C., Fergusson, E., Jenkins, J. and Parr, M. (1997). Attentional biases for emotional faces, *Cognition and Emotion, 11* , 25-42.

Byrne, A. and Eysenck, M.W.(1995).Trait Anxiety, Anxious Mood, and Threat detection. *Cognition and Emotion, 9*, 549-562.

Cacioppo, J.T., and Petty, R.E. (1981). Electromyographic specificity during covert information processing. *Psychophysiology, 18,* 518-523.

Chen, Y. P., Ehlers, A., Clark, D. M., and Mansell, W. (2002). Patients with social phobia direct their attention away from faces. *Behaviour Research and Therapy, 40,* 677-687.

Clark, D.M. (1999). Anxiety disorders: why do they persist and how to treat them. *Behaviour Research and Therapy, 37*, 5-27.

Clark, D.M. and Wells, A. (1995). A Cognitive model of social phobia. In R. Heimberg, M. Liebowitz, D.A. Hope, and F.R. Schneier (Eds), *Social phobia: diagnosis, assessment and treatment.* New York: Guilford Press.

Dimberg, U. (1982). Facial reactions to facial expressions, *Psychophysiology, 19,* 643-647.

Dimberg, U. (1986). Facial expressions as excitatory and inhibitory stimuli for conditioned autonomic responses, *Biological Psychology, 22*, 37-57.

Dimberg, U. (1988). Facial expressions and emotional reactions: A psychobiological analysis of human social behaviour. In H.L. Wagner (Ed), *Social Psychophysiology and Emotion: Theory and Clinical Applications.*(pp131-150). Chichester: Wiley.

Dimberg, U. (1997). Social fear and expressive reactions to social stimuli. *Scandinavian Journal of Psychology, 38*, 171-174.

Dimberg, U., and Thunberg, M. (1998). Rapid facial reactions to emotional facial expressions. *Scandinavian Journal of Psychology, 39*(1), 39-45.

Dimberg, U., Thunberg, M., and Elmehed, K. (2000). Unconscious facial reactions to emotional facial expressions. *Psychological Science, 11*(1), 86-89.

Douilliez, C. and Philippot, P. (2003). Biais dans l'évaluation volontaire de stimuli verbaux et non-verbaux: Effet de l'anxiété sociale. *Revue Francophone de Clinique Comportementale et Cognitive, 8,* 12-18.

Ekman, P. (1971). Universality and cultural differences in facial expressions of emotion. In J.K. Cole (Ed.). *Nebraska Symposium on Motivation* (Vol. 19, pp207-283). Lincoln: University of Nebraska Press.

Ekman, P. (1973). *Darwin and facial expression: a century of research in review.* New-York: Academic Press.

Ekman, P. (1982). *Emotion in the human face* (2nd ed.). Cambridge: Cambridge University Press.

Ekman, P. (1992). An argument for basic emotions, *Cognition and Emotion, 6,* 169-200.

Ekman, P. (1999). Basic emotions. In T. Dalgleish and M.J. Power (Eds), *Handbook of cognition and emotion* (pp. 45-60). Chichester, England: John Wiley and Sons.Ekman, P. and Friesen, W.V. (1975). *Unmasking the face: A guide to recognizing emotions from facial clues.* Englewood Cliffs, NJ: Prentice-Hall.

Ekman, P. and Friesen, W.V. (1975). *Unmasking the face.* A guide to recognizing emotions from facial clues. New Jersey: Prentice Hall Inc.

Ekman, P. and Friesen, W.V. (1978). *The facial action coding system.* Palo Alto, CA: Consulting Psychologists Press.

Esteves, F.(1999). Attentional Bias to emotional Facial Expressions. *European Review of Applied Psychology, 49*, 91-96.

Eysenck, M. W. (1992). *Anxiety: the cognitive perspective.* Hove: Lauwrence Erlbaum Associates.

Foa, E.B., Gilboa-Schechtman, E., Amir, N., Freshman, M. (2000). Memory bias in generalized social phobia: remembering negative emotional expression. *Journal of Anxiety Disorders, 14*, 501-519.

Fox, E. (2002) .Processing emotional facial expressions: The role of anxiety and awareness. *Cognitive, Affective and Behavioral Neuroscience, 2,* 52-63.

Fox, E., Lester, V., Russo, R., Bowles, R.J. , Pichler, A., and Dutton, K. (2000) Facial expressions of emotion: Are angry faces detected more efficiently?. *Cognition-and-Emotion, 14,* 61-92.

Fridlund, A.J. (1994). *Human facial expression: An evolutionary view.* New York: Academic Press.

Gilboa-Schechtman, E., Foa, E.B and Amir, N. (1999). Attentional Biases for Facial Expressions in Social Phobia: The Face-in-the-Crowd Paradigm. *Cognition and Emotion, 13,* 305-318.

Gross, A.L., and Ballif, B. (1991). Children's understanding of emotion from facial expressions and situations: A review. *Developmental Review, 11,* 368-398.

Hansen, C.H. and Hansen, R.D. (1988). Finding the face in the crowd: An anger superiority effect. *Journal of Personality and Social Psychology, 54,* 917-924.

Hampton, C., Purcell, D. G., Bersine, L., Hansen, C. H., and Hansen, R. D. (1989). Probing Pop-out - Another Look at the Face-in-the-Crowd Effect. *Bulletin of the Psychonomic Society, 27*(6), 563-566.

Hess, U., Philippot, P., and Blairy, S., (1999). Mimicry: Fact and Fiction. In P. Philippot, R.S. Feldman, and E.J. Coats (Eds.), *The social context of nonverbal behavior.* (pp. 213-241). New York: Cambridge University Press.

Izard, C.E. (1992). Basic Emotions, relations among emotions, and emotion-cognition relations. *Psychological Review, 99,* 561-565.

Lanzetta, J. T., Cartwright-Smith, J., and Kleck, R. E. (1976). Effect of nonverbal dissimulation on emotional experience and autonomic arousal. *Journal of Personality and Social Psychology,* 33, 354-370.

Lanzetta, J-T. and Orr, S.P. (1980) Influence of facial expressions on the classical conditioning of fear. *Journal of Personality and Social Psychology, 39,* 1081-1087.

Lanzetta, J.T. and Orr, S.P. (1981). Stimulus properties of facial expressions and their influence on the classical conditioning of fear. *Motivation and Emotion, 5,* 225-234.

Levenson, R.W. (1992). Autonomic nervous system differences among emotions. *Psychological Science, 3,* 23-27.

Leventhal, H. (1984). A perceptual-motor theory of emotion. In L. Berkowitz (Ed.), *Advances in Experimental Social Psychology* (Vol. 17, pp. 117-182). New York: Academic Press.

Lundh, L. G. and Ost, L. G. (1996). Recognition bias for critical faces in social phobics. *Behaviour Research and Therapy, 34,* 787-794.

Mac Leod, C. (1990). Mood disorders and cognition. In M.W. Eysenck, *Cognitive Psychology: An International Review.* Chichester: Wiley.

Mac Leod, C. (1999). Anxiety and anxiety disorders. In T. Dalgleish and M.J. Power (Eds.), *Handbook of cognition and emotion* (pp. 447-477). Chichester, England: John Wiley and Sons.

Mac Leod, C. and Mathews, A. (1988).Anxiety and the Allocation of Attention Threat. *The Quarterly Journal of Experimental Psychology,* 40, 651-670.

Mac Leod, C., Mathews, A. and Tata, P. (1986). Attentional Bias in Emotional Disorders. *Journal of Abnormal Psychology, 95,* 15-20.

Mansell, W. (2000). Conscious appraisal and the modification of automatic processes in anxiety. *Behavioural and Cognitive Psychotherapy, 28,* 99-120.

Mansell, W., Clark, D. M., Ehlers, A., and Chen, Y. P. (1999). Social anxiety and attention away from emotional faces. *Cognition and Emotion, 13*, 673-690.

Mathews, A.and Mac Leod, C. (1994).Cognitive approaches to emotion and emotional disorders. *Annual Review of Psychology, 45*, 25-50.

Matsumoto, D. (1992). American-Japanese cultural differences in the recognition of universal facial expressions. *Journal of Cross - Cultural Psychology, 23*, 72-84.

Mc Clure, E.B. and Nowicki, S. (2001). Associations between social anxiety and nonverbal processing skill in preadolescent boys and girls. *Journal of Nonverbal Behavior, 25*, 3-19.

McNally, R.J. (1995). Automaticity and the anxiety disorders. *Behaviour Research and Therapy, 33*, 747-754.

Melfsen, S. and Florin, I. (2002). Do socially anxious children show deficits in classifying facial expressions of emotions? *Journal of Nonverbal Behavior, 26*, 109-126.

Merckelbach, H., Van Hout, W., Van den Hout, M.A. and Mersch, P.P. (1989). Psychophysiological and subjective reactions of social phobics and normals to facial stimuli. *Behaviour Research and Therapy, 27*, 289-294.

Mogg, K. and Braldey, B.P. (1998). A cognitive-motivational analysis of anxiety. *Behavior Research and Therapy, 36,* 809-848.

Mogg, K. and Bradley, B.P. (1999). Orienting attention to threatening facial expressions presented under conditions of restricted awareness. *Cognition and Emotion, 13,* 713-740.

Mogg, K. and Bradley, B.P. (2002). Selective orienting of attention to masked threat faces in social anxiety. *Behaviour Research and Therapy, 40*, 1403-1414.

Mogg, K., Bradley, B. P., de Bono, J. and Painter, M. (1997) Time course of attentional bias for threat information in non-clinical anxiety. *Behaviour Research and Therapy, 35*, 297-303.

Mogg, K., Mathews, A. and Eysenck, M. (1992). Attentional Bias to Threat in Clinical Anxiety States, *Cognition and Emotion, 6,*149-159.

Mogg, K. Philippot, P., and Bradley, B. (2004). Selective attention to angry faces in a clinical sample with social phobia. *Journal of Abnormal Psychology, 113*, 160-165.

Navon, D. and Margalit, B.(1983).Allocation of attention according to informativeness in visual recognition. *The Quarterly Journal of Experimental Psychology,35,* 497-512.

Nelson, C.A. and de Haan, M. (1997). A neurobehavioral approach to the recognition of facial expressions in infancy. In J.A. Russel, and J.M Fernández-Dols (Eds), *The psychology of Facial Expression* (pp. 176-204). New York: Cambridge University Press.

Nothdrurft, H.C. (1993). Faces and facial expressions do not pop out. *Perception, 22*, 1287-1298.

Öhman, A. (1999). Distinguishing unconscious from conscious emotional processes: methodological consideration and theoretical implications. In T. Dalgleish and M.J. Power (Eds.), *Handbook of cognition and emotion* (pp. 765-782). Chichester, England: John Wiley and Sons.

Öhman, A., Dimberg, U., and Öst, L.-G. (1985). Animal and social phobias: biological constraints on learned fear responses. In S. Reiss and R.R. Bootzin (Eds), *Theoretical Issues in Behaviour Therapy.* (pp123-175) New York: Academic Press.

Öhman, A., and Dimberg, U. (1978). Facial expressions as conditionned stimuli for electrodermal responses: a case of preparedness? *Journal of Personality and Social Psychology, 38,* 278-282.

Perez-Lopez, J. R. and Woody, S. R. (2001). Memory for facial expression in social phobia. *Behaviour Research and Therapy, 39*, 967-975.

Philippot, P. (2000). Une approche cognitive de la pathologie des émotions. In Vanderlinden, M. and Danion, J.M. (Eds.), *Neuropsychologie et psychopathologie*. Marseille: Editions Solal.

Philippot, P., Baeyens, C., Douilliez, C., and Francart, B. (2004). Cognitive regulation of emotion. In P. Philippot and R.S. Feldman (Eds.), *The regulation of emotion*. New York: Laurence Erlbaum Associates.

Philippot, P. and Douilliez, C. (2005). Social Phobic do not misinterpret facial expression of emotion. *Behaviour Research and Therapy, 43*, 639-652.

Posner, M.I., Snyder, C.R., and Davidson, B.J. (1980). Attention and the detection of signals. *Journal of Experimental Psychology: General, 109*, 160-174.

Purcell, D.G., Stewart, A.L., and Skov, R.B. (1996). It takes a confounded face to pop out of a crowd, *Perception, 25,* 1091-1108.

Rapee, R.M. and Heimberg, R.G. (1997). A cognitive-behavioral model of anxiety in social phobia. *Behaviour Research and Therapy, 35,* 741-756.

Rosenberg, E.L (1997). The study of Spontaneous Facial Expressions in Psychology. In P. Ekman and E.L. Rosenberg (Eds), *What the face reveals: Basic and applied studies of spontaneous expression using the Facial Action Coding System (FACS).* (pp. 201-216). New York. Oxford University Press.

Russel, J.A. (1994). Is there universal recognition of emotion from facial expression?A review of the cross-cultural studies. In A.J Fridlund. *Human facial expression: An evolutionary view.*(pp192-268). New York: Academic Press.

Russel, J.A. and Fernández-Dols, J.M. (1997). *The psychology of Facial Expression.* New York: Cambridge University Press.

Schwartz, G.E., Fair, P.L., Salt, P., Mandel, M.R., and Klerman, G.L. (1976). Face muscle patterning to affective imagery in depressed and non depressed subjects, *Science, 192*, 489-491.

Seligman, M. (1971). Phobias and preparedness. *Behavior Therapy, 2,* 307-320.

Shiffrin, R.M., and Schneider,W.(1977). Controlled and automatic human information processing: II. Perceptual learning, automatic attending and a general theory. *Psychological-Review, 84*, 127-190.

Spielberger, C.D. (1983). *Manual for the State-Trait Anxiety Inventory.* Palo Alto: Consulting Psychologists Press.

Stemmler, G. (2004). Physiological processes during emotion. In P. Philippot and R. S. Feldman (Eds.), *The regulation of Emotion.* Hillsdale, N.J.: Lauwrence Erlbaum Associates.

Suzuki, S., and Cavanagh, P. (1992). Facial Expression as an Emergent Feature in Visual-Search. *Investigative Ophthalmology and Visual Science, 33*(4), 1355-1355.

Teasdale J.D. (1993). Emotion and two kinds of meaning: Cognitive therapy and applied cognitive science. *Behaviour Research and Therapy, 31*, 339-354.

Teasdale, J.D. (1996). Clinical relevant theory: Integrating clinical insight with cognitive science. In P. Salkovskis (Ed.), Frontiers of cognitive therapy. New York: Guilford.

Watson, D. and Friend, R.(1969). Measurement of social-evaluative anxiety. *Journal of consulting and clinical psychology,33,* 448-457.

Wells, A. and Mathews, G. (1994). *Attention and Emotion: A clinical perspective*. Hove: Lawrence Erlbaum Associates.

White, M.J. (1995). Preattentive analysis of facial expressions of emotion. *Cognition and Emotion, 9*, 439-460.

Williams, J.M.G., Watts, F.N., MacLeod, C. and Mathews, A. (1988). *Cognitive psychology and emotional disorders* . Chichester, U.K.: Wiley.

Winton, E.C., Clark, D.M. and Edelmann, R.J.(1995). Social anxiety, fear of negative evaluation and detection of negative emotion in others. *Behavior Research and Therapy, 33*, 193-196.

Wolfgang, A. and Cohen, M. (1988). Sensitivity of Canadians, Latin Americans, Ethiopians, and Israelis to interracial facial expressions of emotions. *International Journal of Intercultural .relations, 12,* 139-151.

In: Fear in Cognitive Neuroscience
Editor: Salvatore Campanella, pp. 63-95
ISBN: 1-59454-502-2

Chapter 4

THE PERCEPTION OF FEAR IN FACES: INVOLUNTARY AND UNCONSCIOUS RESPONSES IN THE HUMAN BRAIN AS REVEALED BY FUNCTIONAL IMAGING

Gilles Pourtois and Patrik Vuilleumier
Laboratory for behavioral Neurology and Imaging of Cognition, Department of Neuroscience and Clinic of Neurology, University Medical Center, Geneva, Switzerland.
Swiss Center for Affective Sciences, University of Geneva, Geneva, Switzerland

1. INTRODUCTION

1.1. The Concept of Emotion

It has been known for a long time in social sciences that the perception of emotions in con-specifics stands out as one of the most important social skills in human cognition (Darwin, 1872; Frijda, 1989). But until recently in psychology and neurology, the study of emotion has often been left out of the major scope of neuroscience for several different reasons (Damasio, 1994). This situation has substantially evolved over the last decade, and emotion has now become a topic of intense scientific investigation using neuroscience methods. Today, emotions are considered as an essential aspect of cognition in both animals (LeDoux, 1996) and humans (Adolphs, 1999).

However, several debates concerning the place of emotion in human mental life are certainly not settled yet. For instance, does emotion relate to one particular class of cognitive abilities among others, or should emotion and cognition be considered as entirely separate domains (see Ekman and Davidson, 1995)? If so, what are the possible reciprocal influences between emotion and cognitive processes? Such a debate echoes an earlier opposition in psychology during the eighties, between Zajonc's primacy of emotion (1980) and Lazarus's primacy of cognition (1984). New concepts rounded in neurobiological principles are needed to provide a more comprehensive understanding of these complex interrelationships between cognitive and affective processes in human behavior.

Importantly for us here, novel approaches in the study of emotion are now offered by the emergence of Affective Neuroscience, particularly due to the development of brain-imaging techniques. These technical developments have caused a true revolution in neurology and psychology. Since the early nineties, it has indeed become possible to apply sophisticated brain-imaging methods such as Positron Emission Tomography (PET) or functional Magnetic Resonance Imaging (fMRI) to map in vivo specific functions into the human brain, including emotion perception and emotion responses (see Dolan, 2000; Lane and Nadel, 2000). Thus, a growing body of experimental work has been devoted to uncover the functional neuro-anatomy and the neural mechanisms involved in emotion processing (Damasio, 1998), setting the stage for the new field of Affective Neuroscience as a fertile complement to other domains in cognitive neurosciences (Davidson and Sutton, 1995; Panksepp, 1998). This chapter will not provide an exhaustive overview of the literature in Affective Neuroscience, but focus on a subset of brain-imaging data from the research on fear processing. We believe that recent studies have begun to highlight many important aspects related to the functional neuro-anatomy of fear perception, and that these results may provide general principles in order to guide future investigations concerning other emotional systems.

Moreover, we will focus on the evaluative/perceptual aspect of emotion, rather than behavioral responses, emotional expression, or what is known as emotional experience (Lane et al., 1998). In animal research, emotions are defined as internal states produced by instrumental reinforcing stimuli (see Rolls, 1999): emotions are thus synonymous with signals of reward or punishment. In Affective Neuroscience, definitions of emotion are often more sophisticated and do not invoke a unitary construct, but rather a multidimensional one (Clore and Ortony, 2000). Thus, emotion may include (1) physiological changes (including autonomic change), (2) overt behaviors ranging from facial expression to laughter to physical aggression, (3) an internal state that is referred to as affect, and (4) cognitive processes that include thoughts, perceptions, attitudes, and so on (Kolb and Taylor, 2000). Moreover, a basic assumption is that dissociable neural circuits control these different emotionally relevant behaviors. This chapter will emphasize perceptual processing of emotional signals conveyed by faces, and more specifically expressions of fear. Clearly, there is a large variety of different emotional stimuli that might partly implicate the same neural systems, but also seem likely to implicate distinct mechanisms.

1.2. Fear in the Face

The recognition of emotion exhibited by human subjects involves the extraction of a variety of visual (as well as auditory) cues that provide indirect information about these emotional states. Touch and smell may also provide important social signals, but probably to a lesser extent in humans than other mammals. Thus, affective cues can be conveyed through many different channels at the same time (Borod et al., 2000). In the visual modality, affective information is predominantly communicated by the face, but also by body gesture and gait. Within the face channel, different emotions are distinguished through a specialized visual analysis of the face configuration, sensitive to changeable traits but applicable to any individual identity. Other important social visual signals in the face can be communicated by the direction of gaze (see Allison, Puce and McCarthy, 2000), but in this chapter we will mainly review brain imaging experiments investigating facial expressions independently of gaze direction.

In addition, many experiments in psychology and Affective Neurosciences have used non-facial standardized visual stimuli with an emotional content (Lang et al., 1995), for example pictures of snake or spiders to investigate fear perception in humans. However, our review will focus on data obtained by studying fear perception from faces because the latter may constitute a particularly salient and effective biological stimulus in humans (Öhman, 1986), extensively used in various experimental manipulations.

Human subjects share the ability with most other primates to change the configuration of many different facial muscles in order to express and communicate visually several discrete emotions. Some behavioral data (McKelvie, 1995; de Gelder et al., 1997) suggest that the recognition of facial expression is partly based on the face configuration (as opposed to isolated features), e.g. because a comparison of the recognition of facial expressions from upright vs. inverted faces shows a loss of recognition in the latter case. Likewise, configural processing of facial expressions can be demonstrated behaviorally (Calder et al., 2000) using the composite effect (fig.1): composite facial expressions (created by aligning the top half of one expression with the bottom half of another) are harder to identify than non-composite facial expressions (fig. 1), an effect that is independent but parallel to the composite effect found for facial identity (Young et al., 1987).

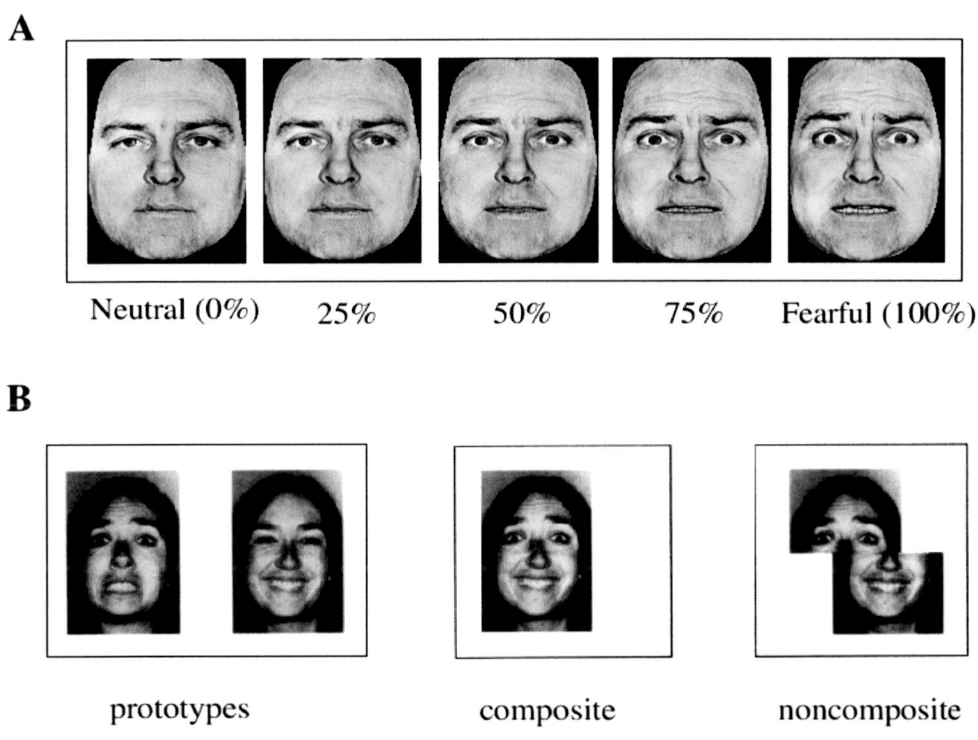

Figure 1. (A) Example of a face continuum Neutral-Fear. The 0% face is the neutral prototype. The 100% face is the prototype for fearful expression. The other intermediate faces were produced by computer graphical manipulation (see section 1.4). (B) Example of composite face expression. The top and bottom segments of two prototype expressions of the same model (left: fear and happy) are combined to create composite (middle) and noncomposite (right) stimuli (Calder et al., 2000).

Face processing is a particularly complex ability enabling us to recognize hundreds of personal identities but only a limited number of expressions. Moreover, it is assumed that we can recognize a face expression correctly without knowing anything about its identity (Bruce and Young, 1986), i.e. irrespective of previous familiarity or knowledge about the person's emotional characteristics. However, emotional expressions tend to be perceived categorically (fig.1; Etcoff and Magee, 1992; Young et al., 1997; Campanella et al., 2002). Such categorical recognition is similar to what is found for phonemes or colors (Harnad, 1987). For instance, behavioral studies have shown that two different faces perceived as reflecting the same emotional category are harder to discriminate apart than two different faces from two different categories (Etcoff and Magee, 1992). This advantage for between-category compared with within-category differences is classically referred as a categorical perception effect (Beale and Keil, 1995; see Campanella et al., 2002 for a recent discussion).

It is traditionally assumed that there exist five or six separate, discrete and basic emotions (Ekman and Friesen, 1976; Ekman, 1992): happiness, sadness, anger, fear, disgust and surprise. The evidence for distinct emotion categories comes from research on facial expressions looking at how human subjects perceive and judge different facial expressions. The typical outcome suggests that basic facial expressions are universal (Ekman, 1992). In other words, there is a high agreement across cultures and races in the labeling of what these expressions signal. We must add that there are also numerous discussions on the role of social or cultural factors that may determine the range of the emotion repertoire or influence the ease of recognition for certain emotions in specific populations. Although our approach is neutral with respect to such issues, the implication of the psychological data is still unclear for the neurobiological results obtained by brain-imaging in healthy subjects who are drawn from different populations (Phelps et al., 2000; Phelps, 2001; Golby et al., 2001).

Many characteristics can be used to distinguish between basic emotions. According to Paul Ekman (1992), one of them is the fact that underlying physiological processes might be specific and that it should be possible to uncover what he called "emotion-specific central nervous system activity". Empirical approaches available from the brain imaging literature have directly addressed the relevance of this assumption, as reviewed in this chapter. Here we concentrate on fear, since it is undoubtedly the emotion that has been studied the most by neuroscience methods (e.g. LeDoux, 1996). In this perspective, fear can be defined in its simplest form as a normal reaction to threatening events (LeDoux, 1996). The animal literature has demonstrated that such reaction to danger or threat seems to be largely hardwired in the brain (Armony and LeDoux, 1996), consistent with the hypothesis of Paul Ekman. Our review will examine to what extent brain imaging in humans has or has not confirmed this strong view of specific emotional modules, e.g. for fear.

To this aim, we first review data indicating that the perception of a fearful face might implicate specialized hardwired systems in the human brain (section 1). Next, we present recent fMRI experiments showing that the neural responses to fearful faces can be observed under some situations where human subjects are not consciously aware of the face stimulus expressing fear (section 2), or not voluntarily attending to it (section 3). These data suggest that some neural responses to fear signals in faces may still take place in a relatively unconscious and automatic way. These aspects provide support to the current view envisaging a modular organization of fear perception (section 4) and a critical role of this fear system in fast adaptive behavior to threats. In addition, these data have also begun to provide new insights on the interrelationships between emotional and perceptual processing that go beyond the strict traditional modular view.

1.3. Methodological Considerations

Physiological measures of human brain function can be derived from Positron Emission Tomography (PET) and functional Magnetic Resonance Imaging (fMRI), which are currently considered as standard tools in cognitive neuroscience. FMRI, the most recent and powerful of these two techniques, allows the visualization of human brain functions with a relatively high spatial resolution. In most human fMRI studies, spatial resolution is usually between 3 and 5 mm in plane with 3-10 mm slice thickness (see Kim, Lee, Goodyear and Silva, 1999). Like all brain imaging techniques, the spatial and temporal resolutions of fMRI are nevertheless limited (see Bandettini, 1999; Kim, Lee, Goodyear and Silva, 1999) and it is important to keep in mind these limitations when looking at results obtained with this technique.

Unlike electro-encephalographic recording, which is a direct measure of integrated local field potential, fMRI offers only an indirect measure of neuronal activity. Functional maps obtained with fMRI are not based on neuronal signals per se but rather reflect the metabolic and heamodynamic changes secondary to neuronal activity. The so-called BOLD (blood oxygenation level-dependent) signal measured in fMRI studies of humans subjects derives from changes in blood oxygenation that occur over a few seconds after the corresponding neural events. Recent data obtained in the monkey brain (Logothetis, Pauls, Augath, Trinath and Oeltermann, 2001) has fortunately confirmed that the coupling between the physiological BOLD response and neuronal activation is tight and well localized, although the response time is relatively slow (in seconds) compared with the time constant of neuronal activity (in tens or hundreds of milliseconds). Furthermore, the data of Logothetis et al. (2001) suggest that activation of an area (as seen by fMRI) predominantly reflects the input to that area and the corresponding local changes in information processing (occurring at the level of post-synaptic dendrites and somata), rather than the output from this area (occurring at the level of the pre-synaptic axons). BOLD responses detected with fMRI correlate well with local field potentials recorded in cortical tissue, depending on the synaptic inputs to a given region more than spiking activity (which reflects the region's output). These data correspond to the fact that the signal to noise ratio for neural signal recorded directly from the brain is much greater than the accompanying fMRI signal. They also suggest that an absence of fMRI signal does not necessarily mean that no information processing is going on in a particular area of the brain (Raichle, 2001), whereas conversely local BOLD responses may provide a reliable index of incoming inputs into associative networks.

Moreover, the signal to noise ratio in fMRI must be high enough in a specific brain region in order to be detected. Unfortunately, this contrast is not absolute or constant across the whole human brain (see Savoy, 2001). Likewise, the signal may fluctuate in time with random white noise, physiological changes, or head motion. Thus, signal to noise ratio in fMRI is also a function of imaging time, sampling rate, field strength, etc. Some methods can increase the signal to noise ratio, such as the use of small surface coil or higher magnetic fields. Nonetheless, the percentage of signal change is often relatively small with standard fMRI, and this is even smaller when event-related designs are used (D'Esposito et al., 1999).

However, event-related designs (where different stimulus types are intermixed) constitute a common and useful experimental procedure. Despite a reduced sensitivity relative to blocked designs (where different stimulus types are given in alternating epochs), fMRI measures related to discrete events seem often preferable to explore the neural bases of fine psychological operations in a more realistic way, including emotion perception.

The dominant methodology used for the analysis of PET and fMRI data in Affective Neuroscience is still largely inspired by the classical assumption of "cognitive subtraction" (Posner et al., 1988). This approach involves a direct comparison between two conditions, subtracting activation evoked by a "control" condition from the activation evoked by another condition of interest, based on the assumption that this contrast will isolate neural processes specifically activated in the latter more than in the former condition. This is a reasonable quantitative assumption, directly inspired by the success of a similar approach used by mental chronometry for reaction time data in cognitive psychology (see Posner, 1978; Posner and Raichle, 1997). However, it remains possible that a difference between two conditions at the level of the brain response (as indexed by the signal change in a given region) is not quantitative but qualitative. In the domain of emotion perception, most of the studies have typically compared brain activations between two emotion categories, usually Fear vs. Neutral (see Breiter et al., 1996) or Fear vs. Happy (see for instance Morris et al., 1996) or sometimes both (see Phillips et al., 1997). In some studies, the authors have also usefully complemented this first subtractive approach by a second method in which they tried to model changes in the functional or effective connectivity between different brain regions (such as the amygdala and the pulvinar, see Morris et al., 1999). This approach (see Friston et al., 1993 for discussions on connectivity based on PET data) also allows going beyond the perspective of isolated neural modules, by providing insights into the dynamical organization of distributed networks.

1.4. Neural Responses to Fearful Faces: A Special Role of the Amygdala

In the literature on emotion processing, the amygdala has a special status and is considered as a key structure in fear processing (Armony and LeDoux, 2000). It is well established based on neurophysiological studies in animals and neuropsychological investigations in humans that fear perception may be particularly disrupted after lesions of this subcortical structure. It was already demonstrated a long time ago that primates with temporal lobe lesions including the amygdala express the Klüver-Bucy syndrome, characterized by enhanced approach behavior, hyperorality, hypersexuality as well as reduced fear (Klüver and Bucy, 1938; Weiskrantz, 1956). However, it remains unclear to what extent the amygdala can also participate to other emotional systems, besides just fear.

In the brain-imaging literature, several researchers since the mid-nineties have provided compelling evidence for a differential neural response of the human amygdala when normal subjects process fearful as opposed to neutral facial expressions, using both PET (Morris et al., 1996) and fMRI (Breiter et al., 1996). This is consistent with neurophysiological recordings in animals, where the amygdala has been found to contain neurons responding selectively to individual faces (see Leonard et al., 1985; Perrett et al., 1992). Many other imaging studies in humans (e.g. investigating threat-related pictures or words, as well as aversive conditioning) have confirmed that fear processing may critically involve the amygdala. This region is now often considered a priori as an anatomical region of interest for statistical analyses when looking at brain responses to threat stimuli (Dolan, 2000).

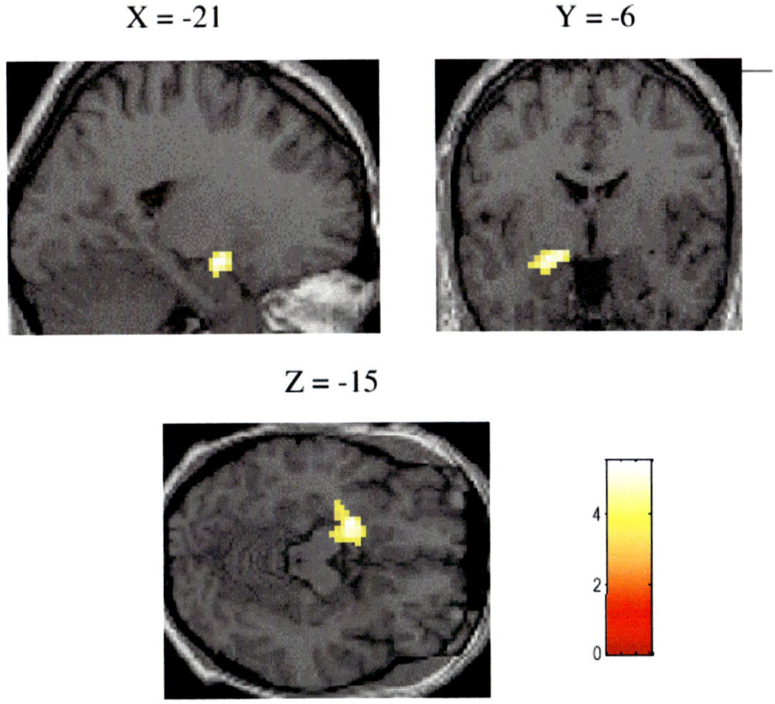

Figure 2. Activation for neutral faces (as contrasted with houses) within the left amygdala of a single normal subject obtained with fMRI (Pourtois and Vuilleumier, unpublished data). This activation (significant at $p < .001$) is superimposed on the structural T1 weighted MRI of the subject which was linearly warped to Talairach space using SPM 99. Talairach coordinates represent; (x) mm lateral to the midline (left = -), (y) mm anterior–posterior to the anterior commissure (posterior = -), and (z) mm inferior–superior to the anterior commissure–posterior commissure plane (inferior = -).

However, the amygdala does not encompass only a single neuronal system (fig.2). In anatomical terms, it refers to a highly differentiated region in the mammalian cerebral hemisphere, located just anterior to the hippocampus in the medial temporal lobe, and composed of a group of at least 13 nuclei or cortical areas. The amygdala receives highly processed sensory information from the anterior temporal lobe (e.g. via cortical pathways that convey visual signals from area V1 through a series of ventral occipitotemporal regions, see Amaral et al., 1992). However, it may also receive direct visual projections from the thalamus (via a subcortical route mediated by the superior colliculus and the pulvinar, see Cowey and Stoerig, 1991; Morris et al., 1999). This subcortical route has been suggested to allow for a rapid evaluation of stimuli with potential threat significance, by-passing detailed analysis in the ventral cortical pathways (e.g. LeDoux, 1996). Outputs of the amygdala include reciprocal projections to the same regions as it receives inputs from, including early sensory visual areas, orbitofrontal cortex, anterior cingulate, ventral striatum, nucleus basalis, and brainstem nuclei. All these regions are implicated in emotional functions.

Within the standard Talairach coordinate system used in neuroimaging (Talairach and Tournoux, 1988), the amygdala has an average width of 15 mm and a slightly longer length.

The amygdala occupies a region that runs from 17 to 30 mm lateral to the midline, 1 mm anterior to 11 mm posterior to the anterior commissure and 7-21 mm below the intercommissural line. It is now clear that fMRI (and PET to a lesser extent) does indeed possess the spatial resolution to image activation foci in the amygdala (see LaBar et al., 2001a for a recent discussion). Some authors have recently argued that fMRI provides a sufficient spatial resolution to image the ventral vs. dorsal division of the human amygdala (Whalen et al., 2001). Moreover, the general location of the amygdala is fairly consistent across subjects (fig.2), allowing comparisons between conditions for group studies (for a recent overview on the functional neuro-anatomy of the amygdala, see Zald, 2003). A particular problem may result in distortion artifacts that are common in this region due to the skull bone density and may require special imaging parameters (see Cordes et al., 2000; Merboldt et al., 2001).

Another notable property of the amygdala is that its heamodynamic changes (as measures with PET or fMRI) associated with responses to emotional events may demonstrate a rapid habituation. The size of the BOLD effect (as measured with fMRI) or rCBF effect (as measured with PET) has often been found to progressively decrease during repeated exposure to emotional stimuli, among which fearful faces (Breiter et al., 1996; Phillips et al., 2001; Wright et al., 2001). In other words, the amygdala tends to respond more during early exposure to emotionally-relevant stimuli, at least under the conditions of typical imaging experiments, but tends to respond less during later repeated exposure. This rapid decline might reflect some ongoing reevaluation of the stimuli that have been exposed previously. This habituation has important consequences for designing a brain-imaging experiment with an interest on the amygdala, as well as for modeling of the expected heamodynamic responses within amygdala.

An early PET study by Morris and collaborators (1996) is particularly informative as to the amygdala sensitivity to signals of fear in faces, because a "morphing" procedure was used to manipulate the intensity of emotion in the faces (fig.1). This procedure consists of a computer graphical manipulation (Benson and Perrett, 1991; Perrett et al., 1994) that can produce different intermediate pictures of faces with graded emotional intensities, between two prototypical expressions (for instance happy and fearful) from the same person identity. In the study of Morris et al. (1996), the morphing procedure was used to shift (by steps of 25%) the facial configuration of the happy face prototype (0%) towards the fear prototype (100%). Three intermediate faces were created between the two extremes based on this algorithm: 25% fear (75 % happy), 50 % fear (50 % happy) and 75 % fear (25 % happy). The results showed that activation of left amygdala increased as a function of the intensity of fearful expression, as did a few other brain regions (left pulvinar, left anterior insula, and the right anterior cingulate cortex). Neural responses to increasing intensity of happy expression were different and included bilateral visual areas in striate cortex, lingual gyrus, and fusiform gyri, as well as the right superior temporal gyrus. Interestingly, neural responses in left amygdala showed a monotonic increase from the most happy to the most fearful expression. This suggests that the amygdala does not only encode changes in category (from happy to fearful) but also changes in intensity (increasing activation with increasing fearfulness).

Since then, many brain-imaging studies have confirmed an involvement of the human amygdala during the processing of fearful faces, across a large variety of tasks. In most of these studies (including Morris et al., 1996), an explicit decision on the face stimuli was required but often did not require judging emotion itself, and emotional processing was thus largely incidental or "implicit" (e.g. one-back repetition, see Dolan and Morris, 2000; gender decision, see Morris et al., 1998a; or identity matching, see Vuilleumier et al., 2001a). An amygdala activation by fearful facial expressions in such circumstances seems consistent with recent findings that its responses may sometimes be independent of visual awareness (section 2) and of selective attention (section 3), as discussed later in this chapter.

1.5. Relation to Visual Awareness

Visual awareness is undoubtedly an important state of human cognition and of our internal representation of the sensory world (Damasio, 1999). Nevertheless, a wide range of studies has revealed that considerable unconscious processing can take place for visual stimuli, sometimes up to fairly elaborate stages of representation. Unconscious visual processes have thus been demonstrated in several cognitive domains including not only perception, but also language, memory, or action control (for overviews see Weiskrantz, 1997; Kohler and Moscovitch, 1997). More recently, in the domain of emotion, researchers have also begun to examine the role of awareness and tested whether conscious awareness is necessary to evoke brain responses during the extraction of emotional significance. Here again, a number of studies using behavioral and functional imaging approaches have concerned the visual processing of fearful faces.

The relation of emotion processing to awareness has also been investigated in patients with focal brain lesions who present with selective deficits in visual awareness. Two major types of brain injury may be responsible for such disorders (see Driver and Mattingley, 1998; Driver and Vuilleumier, 2001). First, patients may show deficient awareness for visual stimuli due to damage to the primary visual cortex in the occipital lobe. If damage is bilateral, the patient suffers from *cortical blindness*, whereas if the lesion is restricted to the primary visual cortex in one hemisphere, the patient has a *hemianopia* (i.e. blindness for stimuli presented in the contralateral visual hemifield) or *quadranopia* (i.e. blindness limited to one quadrant in the contralateral hemifield). In both cases, the scotoma is retinotopic: the blind region can be described according to the retinally corresponding part of the visual field.

Other patients have impaired awareness due to damage to the inferior parietal lobe (or to superior temporal gyrus, see Karnath et al., 2001), particularly in the right hemisphere (Vallar, 1993). In this case, the primary visual cortex may be intact. These patients suffer from *hemispatial neglect*: they show deficient awareness for stimuli in the contralesional (left) side of space, especially in the presence of competing stimuli further to the right (an effect described as "*extinction*"). In the latter case, awareness is preserved for an isolated stimulus on the affected side, but a deficit emerges only when stimuli are presented on both sides simultaneously (Posner, Walker, Friedrich and Rafal, 1984; Baylis, Driver and Rafal, 1993). Unlike cortical blindness or hemianopia due to damage to the primary visual cortex, the loss of conscious perception in spatial neglect and extinction cannot be described in retinal coordinates, i.e. it is not purely retinotopic. It is commonly assumed that an impairment in *spatial attention* plays an essential role in neglect and extinction (Driver and Vuilleumier, 2001; Tong, 2003), unlike the primary damage to more basic mechanisms of conscious visual perception associated with cortical blindness (see also Kentridge, Heywood and Weiskrantz, 1999).

An intriguing finding provided by the study of patients with disturbances in visual awareness (either due to neglect/extinction or hemianopia/blindsight) is that some unconscious processing appears still to take place for fearful faces when these are presented in a part of the visual field or visual space where the patients have no awareness of the stimulus occurrence. The following two sections will consider recent brain-imaging data related to this point, providing evidence for differential brain responses to fearful faces under conditions of reduced visual awareness of these faces (due to backward masking or cortical blindness, see section 2) or under conditions of reduced visual attention (due to the demands of an additional task or to parietal neglect, see section 3).

2. The Role of Visual Awareness

2.1. Backward Masking

In the laboratory as well as in the scanner, it is possible to experimentally manipulate awareness of visual stimuli and thus explore whether it is a necessary condition to yield a given cognitive process (e.g. the perception of fear from a face). Psychologists and neurologists have developed several methods to investigate in normal observers to what extent cognitive processes can still take place when conscious vision is absent or highly reduced. A commonly used approach is the backward masking method (Breitmeyer, 1984; Macknik and Livingstone, 1998).

Backward visual masking is a powerful manipulation to yield subliminal presentation of a target stimulus. The target stimulus (e.g. a fearful face) is briefly presented (typically for less than 40 ms) and then directly masked by a second visual stimulus (e.g. a neutral face) usually presented for a longer time than the target stimulus (e.g. 200 ms) and called the mask. Importantly, the offset of the target stimulus must coincide with the onset of the mask. Using this trick, typically, almost all participants only report the mask and do not see "consciously" the target stimulus as demonstrated by objective forced-choice tasks and subjective reports. In other words, awareness of the target is highly reduced. Backward masking can of course be employed to investigate subliminal processing of various types of stimuli (see Macknik and Livingstone, 1998).

When looking at brain activation during backward masking experiments using faces (Whalen et al., 1998; Morris et al., 1998a), fMRI studies have demonstrated significant amygdala responses during masked exposure to fearful facial expressions. In the fMRI study by Whalen et al. (1998), a significant decrease was also observed within the amygdala in response to masked happy faces, consistent with the notion that the level of amygdala activation is differentially affected by the emotional valence of the target stimulus. These results have been subsequently replicated in similar paradigms (see Rauch et al., 2000), and with masked faces that had been conditioned by pairing with an aversive sound stimulus (Critchley et al., 2002).

2.2. Classical Fear Conditioning

Conditioning is a basic form of associative learning (Pavlov, 1927), whereby a neutral stimulus (for instance a neutral face) acquires behavioral significance through its temporal pairing with an innately salient unconditioned stimulus (for instance a loud white noise). Importantly, the conditioning contingency is unknown to the subjects: for instance, they may perform an irrelevant task on the neutral stimuli while the latter acquire an affective salience through their systematic (although often unnoticed) pairing with the unconditioned stimulus. This simple but powerful form of learning has made it possible to explore the functional neuro-anatomy involved in the acquisition/conditioning of fear responses.

Fear or aversive conditioning has been successfully adapted in several brain-imaging studies in humans (Dolan and Morris, 2000; LaBar et al., 1998). A typical procedure was as follows. Prior to scanning, subjects were exposed to faces (happy, fearful or neutral) that could be either paired with a noise stimulus (CS+) or remained unpaired (CS-). At the end of the conditioning period, and therefore at the start of the extinction period, subjects were scanned using PET (Dolan and Morris, 2000). In half of the scans, faces that had been paired with noise were presented and in the other half, faces that had remained unpaired were presented. Noises were never played during this extinction phase.

The comparison of brain activation in response to the CS+ versus CS- condition (across all types of faces) revealed differential activations in a number of brain regions, all in the right hemisphere: orbitofrontal cortex, superior frontal gyrus, pulvinar, and reticular nuclei of the thalamus. When looking at brain regions activated by learned fear responses specifically to happy faces, activation in the right pulvinar was also found. Importantly, such activity in the pulvinar was a good predictor of concomitant activation of different cortical and subcortical regions among which the right amygdala, indicating significant "functional coupling" between these regions. These results are consistent with the notion that the pulvinar may play a crucial role in the coordination of neural processing in sensory and association cortices (see Olshausen et al., 1993). More importantly, these data show that when subjects have acquired, through conditioning, a fear response to previously non-fearful faces, activation is seen in both the right amygdala and connected areas. Another imaging study (LaBar et al., 1998) using fear conditioning with non-facial stimuli found a similar activation of the amygdala to the CS+ stimuli. Altogether, these brain-imaging data are compatible with behavioral studies in animals and brain-damaged patients indicating an important role of the amygdala in emotional learning (LeDoux, 1996; LaBar et al., 1995), and extensive connections between amygdala and other brain regions (LeDoux, 1996; Amaral et al., 1992).

Although in this situation the conditioning association is entirely unknown to subjects (i.e. subjects remain "blind" to the pairing contingency), they are nonetheless fully aware of the visual stimulus that acquires a new salience through conditioning. However, is awareness of the visual stimulus a necessary condition to observe an activation of the amygdala and related structures during fear conditioning? Based on behavioral studies, we know that an aversively conditioned masked stimulus can elicit an emotional response (such as measure in the galvanic skin conductance response) even when subjects do not see consciously the stimulus (Esteves and Öhman, 1993; Esteves et al., 1994). This question about the role of stimulus awareness has also been addressed in several brain-imaging experiments. These studies have further confirmed a major role of the amygdala and pulvinar in fear conditioning.

Again, awareness of face stimuli was manipulated using a backward visual masking method (see section 2.1), where a given face (with an angry expression) acquired salience through aversive conditioning due to its systematic pairing with a burst of white noise (Morris et al., 1998). During the acquisition phase, the angry face (CS+) was backwardly masked with a neutral face. Using PET, Morris et al. (1998b) compared masked vs. unmasked presentations of the conditioned angry face and found significant activation in the right amygdala. The reverse contrast showed significant activation in the left amygdala. These results support an involvement of the amygdala in classical fear conditioning, and in addition suggest a lateralized response according to the level of awareness. Right amygdala appeared to respond to the affective value of the CS+ more specifically when subjects were unaware of the face, whereas conversely left amygdala responded more when subjects were aware of the face. Furthermore, an analysis testing the functional connectivity between brain regions, across these different stimulus conditions, found additional evidence for an increased coupling between right amygdala, pulvinar and superior colliculus specifically when subjects viewed masked fear-conditioned faces. These results have been subsequently extended using fMRI (Morris et al., 2001a). This coupling has been interpreted as reflecting an involvement of subcortical visual pathways during detection of threat-related cues in faces in the absence of conscious visual awareness. Moreover, the amygdala was also found to be activated by masked faces with fearful expressions (compared to neutral or happy) even without prior associative conditioning and without explicit awareness of these faces (Whalen et al., 1998).

2.3. Blindsight

Blind patients with striate cortex lesions may still exhibit some residual visual abilities which can be revealed using fine psychophysical tests, a phenomenon referred to as "blindsight" (Poppel et al., 1973; Weiskrantz et al., 1974; see Weiskrantz, 1986, 1997). Thus, these patients can make accurate guesses about the attributes of stimuli presented to their blind field (e.g. simple presence, orientation, motion, etc.) even though they have no conscious perception of the stimulus. This provides a very interesting situation for psychologists and neurologists to investigate the role of awareness in cognitive processes, and the nature of operations that can proceed without awareness, such as the perception of fearful faces.

Behavioral studies with blindsight patients have reported various forms of unconscious processing for elementary visual stimuli. These patients can discriminate the presence, location, orientation, wavelength, and direction of movement of a target stimulus above chance level despite reporting no awareness of the stimulus. More recently, both behavioral and brain-imaging data obtained with two blindsight patients (GY and DB) has also suggested the existence of some unaware residual visual ability for the recognition of facial expressions (fig.3), a phenomenon called "affective blindsight" (see de Gelder et al., 1999, 2001, 2002; Weiskrantz, 2000; Hamm et al., 2003).

GY is a 45 years old male who sustained damage to the posterior left hemisphere of his brain by head injury (a road accident) when he was 7 years old (fig.3). Consequently, GY suffers from a right hemianopia. Based on measures of the patient's forced-choice guesses, GY can still discriminate above chance different facial expressions (sad, anger, fear and happiness) when these are presented in his blind visual hemifield (de Gelder et al., 1999). These behavioral results in GY have been subsequently replicated with a second blindsight patient (DB). DB is a 61 years old male in whom an arterious venous malformation in the medial right occipital lobe was surgically removed when he was 33 years old. Consequently, DB suffers from a left hemianopia. Data from these two patients suggest that residual "affective blindsight" may be independent of the hemispheric side of visual cortical lesions.

A

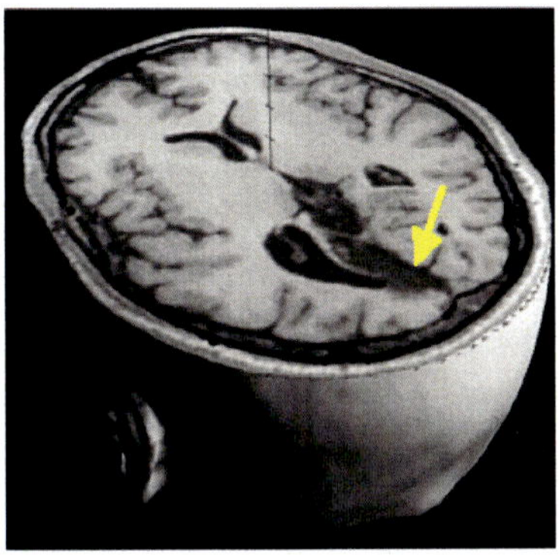

B

Stimuli	Response			
	Happy	Sad	Angry	Fearful
Happy	27	2	6	1
Sad	1	24	5	6
Angry	3	11	13	9
Fearful	2	12	6	15

Figure 3. (A) 3D structural MRI of GY's brain (posterior view). The arrow indicates the location and extent of the lesion in the left occipital lobe including V1 (Morris et al., 2001b). (B) Behavioral performance of GY (confusion matrix of responses to happy, sad, angry and fearful faces) indicating some residual visual abilities (correct guesses) to discriminate among different facial expressions when these face stimuli were directly presented in his blind (right) visual field (de Gelder et al., 1999).

It is commonly assumed that measures of forced-choice guesses cannot unambiguously establish a "blindsight" phenomenon because they leave open the possibility of deliberate response strategy (see Azzopardi and Cowey, 1998 for a discussion). Therefore, in a follow-up study (de Gelder et al., 2001), GY was again tested for his residual visual abilities using an indirect method inspired from studies with right-parietal brain-damaged patient with left spatial neglect and visual extinction (see section 3). This indirect method consists of investigating recognition of facial expressions in the intact visual field depending on simultaneous presentation of congruent or incongruent face stimuli in the blind field. With GY, results showed that redundant stimulation in the blind field led to shorter latencies for stimulus recognition in the intact field (de Gelder et al., 2001). Again, this effect was not restricted to fearful faces but extended to other emotion categories (e.g. happy expressions).

Consistent with these behavioural results, a subsequent fMRI study (Morris et al., 2001b) reported that amygdala responses were still evoked in the blindsight patient GY during the presentation of either fearful faces or fear-conditioned faces in the blind hemifield. These results suggest a role of subcortical inputs (probably mediated by the superior colliculus and the pulvinar, see Cowey and Stoerig, 1991) that are susceptible to reach the amygdala via a route that bypasses the lesioned striate cortex. These brain-imaging data therefore converge with previous neuroimaging studies reviewed above that have shown amygdala activation to unseen (backward masked) emotional stimuli in neurologically intact subjects, and similarly suggested a role of subcortical visual inputs to the amygdala.

2.4. Unseen Fear in the Brain

We have reviewed different brain-imaging data that all suggest that stimulus awareness is not always necessary to observe differential brain responses to fearful faces, particularly within the amygdala. Although visual awareness is a complex mental state (Baars, 1988; Damasio, 1999; Tong, 2003), it can be manipulated using specific experimental manipulations in normal observers (such as backward masking or classical conditioning) or even more radically by taking advantage of focal brain lesions in humans. In this latter case, behavioral and brain-imaging data indicate that patients with damage to the striate cortex can still show "blindsight" for emotional faces. Such unconscious processing of emotion in humans would appear consistent with findings in animals showing that fear responses can be obtained in the amygdala even during deep anaesthesia (Rosenkrantz and Grace, 2002), where awareness is profoundly suppressed. Altogether, these results suggest that at least some fear-relevant signals might be susceptible to reach the amygdala via a route that bypasses elaborate processing in the primary visual cortex, and perhaps involves a subcortical colliculo-thalamic route parallel to the cortical geniculo-striate pathway (Cowey and Stoerig, 1991; see Lamme, 2001 for a recent review). However, the nature and extent of processing mediated by this subcortical route is still relatively debated and remains to be more clearly specified. Alternative routes might also exist within other pathways, including from superior colliculus to V2, pulvinar to inferior temporal cortex, or cortical connections to STS.

Hence, even though fearful faces selectively activate the amygdala under conditions where conscious vision is absent or at least strongly reduced, it does not necessarily imply that all aspects of fear processing are unconscious and exclusively processed within the amygdala (see Barbur et al., 1993 for a similar discussion on the role of area V5 in the conscious vs. unconscious perception of visual motion). Several fMRI studies reviewed here also indicated that activation to fearful faces in other cortical regions (e.g. fusiform and orbitofrontal) might depend on awareness of the visual stimuli (see Whalen et al., 1998; Morris et al., 1999, 2001b). In the PET study of Morris et al. (1999), a dissociation was even found between the left and right amygdala: the activity of the former was not different between seen vs. unseen fear-conditioned targets whereas that of the latter was specifically related with the pulvinar and superior colliculus in the unseen condition. It remains to establish which components or aspects of fearful signal can be processed unconsciously and which ones require conscious vision. For instance, recent fMRI data (Vuilleumier et al., 2003) indicate that low-spatial frequencies (as opposed to high spatial frequencies) contained in fearful faces may activate a network of subcortial regions, including the pulvinar, the amygdala and the superior colliculus, which might be preferentially involved in the non-conscious processing of these relevant visual stimuli (Morris et al., 1999). Similar questions have been raised for the role of selective visual attention in the perception of fearful faces. In the next section, we will consider recent brain-imaging data that have directly addressed this issue.

3. The Role of Selective Visual Attention

3.1. Extinction and Neglect

We have already mentioned above that visual attention is disrupted in hemispatial neglect, which often occurs after a stroke in the inferior posterior parietal cortex of the right hemisphere (Vallar, 1993; Driver and Vuilleumier, 2001). Perceptual extinction is a frequent phenomenon in patients who have neglect, which cannot be explained by elementary sensory defects (i.e. blindness) since these patients may report a stimulus in their contralesional (e.g. left) visual field presented alone, but typically remain unaware of the same stimulus when attention is captured by another competing stimulus in the ipsilesional (e.g. right) visual field (for a recent review, see Driver and Vuilleumier, 2001). In these patients, visual cortical pathways from occipital to temporal lobe may be entirely spared by the lesion, including amygdala regions.

Behavioral results in patients with neglect and extinction indicate that their visual awareness of contralesional stimuli can be modulated according to the emotional valence of these stimuli. Thus, severity of perceptual extinction is less severe for faces with emotional expressions (happy or angry) than for neutral faces (Vuilleumier and Schwartz, 2001a), and less severe for emotional pictures (spiders) than for neutral pictures (flowers) with the same visual complexity (Vuilleumier and Schwartz, 2001b). These effects imply that emotion can be extracted from the contralesional inputs under conditions where spatial attention tends to be pathologically captured by competing stimuli on the ipsilesional side, but also that the detection of emotion signals can partly reverse this deficit in spatial attention, hence reducing perceptual extinction (see Vuilleumier, 2002). Moreover, this effect in neglect patients does not seem to be specific to fear, neither to fearful faces, an observation that we have already noticed above with blindsight patients (section 2.3).

These findings are consistent with previous results in normal viewers (see Vuilleumier, 2002). Several behavioral experiments using visual search paradigms in healthy subjects have provided evidence for a more rapid detection of faces with negative (and to a lesser degree, also positive) expressions among neutral distracters (Eastwood et al., 2001; Hansen and Hansen, 1988; Öhman et al., 2001), than vice versa. This advantage is usually expressed as a smaller cost of the number of distracters on visual search efficiency (i.e. the search slope is shallower for emotional versus neutral stimuli, though not necessarily flat as during "pop-out" for elementary visual features). Overall, these results suggest that some mechanisms may facilitate the detection of emotional stimuli at an early stage of visual processing (prior to stages where attentive search can operate; see Treisman and Gelade, 1980). The most consistent capture of attention by emotion in these search conditions is usually found with negatively valenced or fear-related stimuli (Öhman et al., 2000), unlike an equal advantage found for both angry and happy faces in neglect (Vuilleumier and Schwartz, 2001b). Moreover, such effects of emotion on visual perception and attention in healthy subjects may be modulated by individual differences in anxiety traits (see Mogg et al., 2000; Fox, 2002). It remains to be determined whether such predisposition factors are also relevant in brain-damaged patients.

3.2. Partial Independence Between Attention and Emotion

In the previous sections, we have presented data indicating that the perception of fearful faces activates specific brain regions, including not only the amygdala but also face-sensitive visual cortical areas in the fusiform gyrus. An important question given behavioral evidence of emotional processing prior to attentional selection is whether these differential neural responses to fear are modulated by selective visual attention or not. Indeed, there is good evidence that activation in a number of cortical and even subcortical regions can be modulated by attention (see Kastner and Ungerleider, 2000; Corbetta and Shulman, 2002 for recent overviews). To date, this question has been addressed only by a few brain-imaging studies, using different manipulations of attention.

A number of investigators compared neural responses to emotional faces during incidental or "implicit" processing of emotion (i.e. when facial expression is irrelevant to the task, e.g. during gender discrimination), versus "explicit" processing of emotion (i.e. when the task requires judging facial expression). A general finding is that some brain regions respond to emotion only when it is task-relevant, including the temporal lobe cortex (such as superior temporal sulcus), right frontal cortex, and insular cortex (Critchley et al., 2000; Gorno-Tempini et al., 2001; Naramuto et al., 2001), whereas other regions (e.g. left inferior frontal cortex, bilateral occipito-temporal junction) may respond to emotion irrespective of the task. In particular, the latter pattern was found in the amygdala for happy and angry faces (Critchley et al., 2000), although not for stimuli with less of an intrinsic biological significance (Keightley et al., 2000). Moreover, a modulation of amygdala responses as a function of task was reported in a few studies, but where the task was potentially confounded with changes in the stimuli (Hariri et al., 2000).

Three recent fMRI studies, in normal observers (Vuilleumier et al., 2001a; Pessoa et al., 2003) and in a neglect patient (Vuilleumier et al., 2002, see also Vuilleumier et al., 2001b), have directly explored the role of spatial attention on the processing of fearful faces. Some results from these studies suggest that a response to fearful faces can still arise regardless of voluntary spatial attention. In an event-related fMRI study (Vuilleumier et al., 2001a), normal viewers were presented with stimulus arrays containing two faces and two non-face stimuli (houses) appearing at eccentric locations (fig.4). Subjects fixated a central point and were instructed to covertly focus their attention on two eccentric locations and to match the two stimuli at these locations (i.e. judge whether faces were the same or different, or whether houses were the same or different), while ignoring the stimuli at the two other locations. In addition, expression of the faces was either fearful or neutral, regardless of whether attention was focused on the face pairs or on the house pairs. All trial types were fully randomized. In this design, therefore, neural response to fearful emotional expression could directly be compared for faces in the focus of attention and faces outside the focus of attention.

A first result was that spatial attention strongly modulated activity in extrastriate visual areas, with increased responses in bilateral fusiform cortex when faces appeared at the relevant locations and increased activity in parahippocampal cortex when houses appeared at the relevant locations. This is consistent with previous studies (Corbetta and Shulman, 2002, Wojciulik et al., 1998) showing a robust modulation of visual cortex by attention. More importantly, the results also revealed that a response to fearful faces occurred in the left amygdala (as well as the face fusiform area) regardless of whether the faces were presented at the task-relevant or irrelevant locations, suggesting that these emotional responses were largely independent of the modulation by spatial attention observed in extrastriate visual cortex (fig.4). This converges with behavioral results reviewed above suggesting that emotional significance can be extracted from stimuli outside the current focus of attention (for a review, see Vuilleumier, 2002; Vuilleumier et al., 2004).

By contrast, an effect of spatial attention on the responses to fearful faces (i.e. an increased activation by fear specifically when the faces appeared at the relevant locations) was found in the striate cortex, medial temporal pole, and caudal parts of the anterior cingulate cortex (all in the left hemisphere) (Vuilleumier et al., 2001a), whereas other results suggested even more widespread influences of attention during a different task (Pessoa et al., 2002).

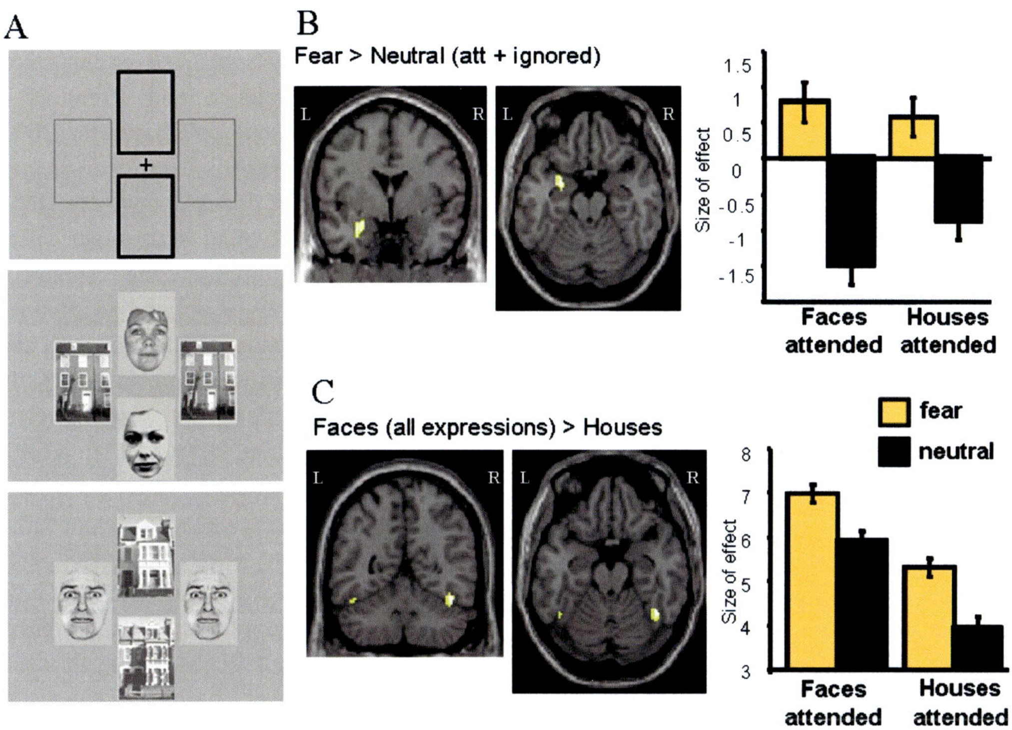

Figure 4. (A) Displays with one pair of faces and one pair of houses arranged at orthogonal position, briefly presented on each trial during fMRI scanning. Faces had either a neutral or fearful expression. Prior to stimulus presentation, subjects were cued to either the two vertical or the two horizontal stimuli and asked to perform a matching task (same or different judgments) for the stimulus pair at the cued locations. (B) fMRI results showing an activation within the left amygdala to fearful compared to neutral faces that is similar when faces are task-relevant vs. irrelevant, i.e., inside vs. outside the attentional focus (Vuilleumier et al., 2001a). (C) By contrast, activation of the face-selective areas in fusiform cortex was strongly modulated by spatial attention, with significant increases when faces were task-relevant.

Similar results were obtained by an event-related fMRI study of a right-parietal brain-damaged patient with left spatial neglect and visual extinction (Vuilleumier et al., 2002). Pictures of fearful faces, neutral faces, or houses were briefly presented either in his intact right visual field, in the neglected left visual field, or in both fields simultaneously. In the latter critical type of trial, a face with either a fearful or neutral expression appeared on the left side together with a house on the right side, with the left face being extinguished from the

4. Conclusions

4.1. Modularity

Recent research in Affective Neuroscience and brain-imaging has emphasized the critical role of a "fear module" centered on the amygdala (LeDoux, 1996; Öhman et al., 2000). At the first glance, several aspects in the data reviewed in this chapter would appear consistent with this modular view, particularly the findings that unconscious and involuntary responses to fear may be evoked in the amygdala through hardwired and autonomous circuits in the brain.

Modularity is an important but controversial concept in cognitive sciences. Modularity means that the cognitive system is composed of functional components, whose operation can be characterized independently of the functions of other components, and that these components can be selectively impaired by brain damage (Fodor, 1983). Although often questioned (see Fuster, 2000), modularity has also been proposed at the level of brain organization itself. Thus, cognitive organization in the cortex may be viewed as a hierarchical assembly of specialized cortical modules (i.e. with a discrete and contiguous piece of cortical tissue dedicated to serve one specific cognitive function or to represent one specific aspect of information). This conception is still very common in cognitive neuroscience but also in affective neuroscience. For instance, in terms of neural architecture, it has been proposed that the ventral temporal cortex may contain a limited number of areas that are specialized for representing specific categories of stimuli, such as the fusiform area for faces (FFA) and the parahippocampal area for places (PPA). However this issue is far from being settled (see for example Kanwisher et al., 1997; Kanwisher, 2000 but also Tarr and Gauthier, 2000; Haxby et al., 2000).

In Fodor's conception, a module can be characterized by a list of functional properties: it is domain-specific, innately specified, informationally encapsulated, efficient, hard-wired (neural specific), autonomous, and not assembled. Nowadays, domain-specificity (i.e. the module is not responding to inputs other than those of a particular "class") is often considered as the crucial argument to test for modularity at the empirical level (Coltheart, 1999).

In this chapter, we have presented brain-imaging data suggesting that the perception of fearful faces selectively engages the amygdala, sometimes in relatively obligatory manner, apparently supporting the view that the amygdala might constitute a specialized module for threat detection. Indeed, in many situations, neural responses within the amygdala may be characterized as unconscious and automatic since such responses are evoked even though subjects are not aware of the fearful faces or not attending to them. These data are therefore partly consistent with the notion of a cerebral module for fear perception, centered on the amygdala. However, a strict modular perspective should be questioned by a careful analysis of the degree of executive control and attentional modulation that can be exerted on amygdala activity (e.g. Phelps et al., 2002; Pessoa et al., 2002), as well as by the complex and reciprocal interactions that can take place between the amygdala and many distant interconnected regions, such as the fusiform cortex, frontal cortex, or subcortical thalamic nuclei.

4.2. Explicit vs. Implicit Processes

A recurrent theme in the brain-imaging data reviewed in this chapter suggests that the recognition of fearful facial expressions may be involuntary ("automatic") and implicit (without explicit intention to evaluate emotion). This distinction between implicit vs. explicit processes is fundamental in cognitive neurosciences, but also controversial. Implicit processing has been found in many domains such as memory, language, perception or motor control (for overviews see Weiskrantz, 1997; Kohler and Moscovitch, 1997). Here, we have noted that discriminative brain responses to fearful facial expressions may be generated outside the scope of conscious awareness and without selective visual attention. In other words, several brain-imaging results suggest that the recognition of fearful facial expressions can be "implicit" under these circumstances, although it remains to be determined whether the cognitive context, expectation, or degree of arousal evoked by conscious perception of stimuli during a given task may or may not influence the observed responsiveness to emotional stimuli during implicit and unconscious conditions.

In this perspective, it is relevant to recall that several fMRI studies (e.g. Critchley et al., 2000; Gorno-Tempini et al., 2001) compared intentional ("explicit") and incidental ("implicit") processing of emotional faces. Emotional responses in medial temporal limbic regions (such as amygdala) independent of task goals have been more consistently reported for fearful or negative faces, whereas task-dependent responses have usually been found for other expressions (see Vuilleumier, 2002 for a recent review). Again, this would be consistent with a special status of fear-related processing in the amygdala (Öhman and Mineka, 2001).

4.3. Face Recognition as a Module

In this chapter, we have focused on fear perception when this emotion is conveyed by facial expression. In itself, face recognition has also often been thought to be modular, subserved by specialized and localized cortical areas in the fusiform gyrus (for discussion and controversies, see Kanwisher, 2000 and Tarr and Gauthier, 2000). Within this model, the fusiform gyrus is involved in processing the structural properties of the faces that are reliable indicators of personal identity, whereas regions more anterior and dorsal in the temporal lobe (e.g. the superior temporal sulcus and gyrus) are involved in processing information about the changeable configurations of face (e.g. facial expression, eye movement, lip reading...).

However, recent fMRI data (Haxby, Gobbini, Furey, Ishai, Schouten, and Pietrini, 2001) suggest that even if a modular specialization may exist in the human brain for face recognition, the organization of visual object representations is potentially more sophisticated and distributed, than simply localized in a unique region of ventral temporal cortex for a given category. Face perception may engage several different regions at the same time, not only fusiform cortex but also lateral occipital areas, superior temporal sulcus, frontal areas, as well as amygdala (Haxby et al., 2000). Thus, the neural representation of any individual face might not unequivocally be imputed to only a single area in the brain, but rather involve a distributed assembly of neurons coding distinct aspects of facial information (but see Spiridon and Kanwisher, 2002 for an opposite view). Moreover, brain-imaging findings in humans (Morris et al., 1998b; Vuilleumier et al., 2001a) as well as single cell recordings in monkeys (Sugase et al., 1999) have shown that neural responses in face-sensitive areas or face-selective neurons, respectively, can be modulated by the emotional expression of faces, even when such expression is irrelevant to the current task, suggesting that some feedback influences may be exerted by amygdala or other regions processing emotion onto the cortical regions analyzing face identity traits. Such effects reveal significant reciprocal interactions between the proposed "modules".

4.4. Which Module for Fear Perception?

A number of behavioral studies in human subjects have also concluded that recognition of fear from the face is automatic (Öhman et al., 1999) and rapidly manifested after birth (Nelson et al., 1979; Nelson and Dolgin, 1985). Based on neurospychological studies of patients with amygdala damage who show selective deficits in the recognition of fearful facial expressions (Adolphs et al., 1994; see Calder et al., 2001) and in fear conditioning (Bechara et al., 1995, LaBar et al., 1995), plus some electrophysiological results (Halgren et al., 1978) and imaging results in healthy humans (Morris et al., 1996, Whalen et al., 1998, LaBar et al., 1998, Buchel and Dolan, 2000), behavioral data might also be taken to suggest that the amygdala may constitute a key structure responsible for fear processing in an automatic and modular way (e.g. Öhman and Mineka, 2001). Within this model, fear (not necessarily restricted to faces) might have a special status compared with other emotion categories.

However, an implementation of the inputs to an amygdala fear module would mean that cognitive penetrability of this system is limited. Although a number brain-imaging results can be interpreted in support of this modular view (e.g. with emotional responses to faces being independent of voluntary attentional control and awareness of the stimulus), it is worth emphasizing that other data are not entirely consistent with a strict modular view.

First, the vast majority of brain imaging experiments on emotion perception clearly show that the amygdala is not the only brain structure activated by fear, or by related emotions. For instance, the ventral striatum and orbitofrontal cortex are other important brain regions concerned by emotional responses, possibly critically involved in associating a perceptual representation with affective significance. Ventro-lateral frontal regions and superior temporal sulcus are also implicated in the analysis of facial emotional expression (Haxby et al., 2000, Sprengelmeyer et al., 1998). However, these latter areas are often activated by other categories of facial expression, suggesting a more general function in emotional behavior rather than just the perceptual processing of facial signals of fear (see Vuilleumier et al., 2004). Their exact contribution to affective processing and affective experience remains to be determined.

Second, the amygdala has sometimes been found to be activated by faces with other negative expressions (see Zald, 2003 for a recent overview) such as anger (Critchley et al., 2000; Whalen et al., 2001) or sadness (Blair et al., 1999), or even by happy but arousing stimuli (Lane et al., 1997). In addition, a recent fMRI study showed the involvement of the amygdala in response to neutral faces perceived as "untrustworthy" through subjective ratings (Winston et al., 2002). This is also hardly compatible with a strict modular conception of fear processing, sensitive only to a very specific class of inputs. In the same vein, the amygdala is known to be activated by fear signals presented in non-visual sensory channels, such as voices (Phillips et al., 1998), or presented concurrently in both the visual and auditory modalities (Dolan et al., 2001). Responses to complex visual scenes (Irwin et al., 1996;

Taylor et al., 1998; Hariri et al., 2002) or words (Tabert et al., 2001) have also been reported. A more general role for the amygdala than just in fear processing is indicated by the recent findings of activation by perceived eye gaze contact (Kawashima et al., 1999; George et al., 2001; Morris et al., 2002). In the same perspective, some brain-imaging data (Wright et al., 2003) also indicate that the amygdala, together with other brain regions (e.g. substantia innominata), might actually be implicated in novelty detection rather than just the processing of fearful faces. These data show that novel (as opposed to repeated) neutral faces activate the amygdala whereas the inferior temporal cortex shows a different response profile. The amygdala could also be involved in vigilance reactions to ambiguous stimuli: PET data indicate that the (left) amygdala activates to unusual photographs as contrasted with uninteresting neutral photographs (Hamann et al., 2002). These data conform to the proposal that the amygdala would be involved in increasing vigilance and attention based on stimulus ambiguity (Whalen et al., 2001). This range of effective stimuli clearly suggests that appropriate inputs to the amygdala may implicate fairly complex and flexible representations, going far beyond the mere perception of fearful faces.

Third, there are compelling data demonstrating that under certain circumstances the amygdala may partly be penetrable by higher order beliefs (Phelps et al., 2001) or by expectations of cognitive choices and decisions (Kahn et al., 2002). In this context, Phelps and colleagues (2001) provided evidence that the human amygdala is not strictly encapsulated. They used an instructed fear paradigm in which subjects learned that an event was associated to an aversive outcome. Importantly, this aversive outcome never happened but was only evoked through verbal communication. Results also suggested that this symbolic representation of fear was conveyed to the amygdala through the insular cortex. Similarly, LaBar and colleagues (2001b) have shown that the amygdala was more activated by the visual presentation of food-related stimuli when participants were in a hungry state than when they were in a satiated state, which complicates again a strict modular view of amygdala function. In addition, it remains to clarify to what extent amygdala responsiveness may be determined or modulated by other factors such as selective attention (Pessoa et al., 2002), task-related set (Hariri et al., 2000), general arousal (Williams et al., 2001), or individual personality factors (Canli et al., 2002; Hariri et al., 2002; Schwartz et al., 2003).

To resume, it seems reasonable to argue that amygdala activation revealed by brain-imaging experiments may not only be linked to the perception of fearful faces but more likely reflect a broader role in processing and learning about relevant social and motivational signals in the environment. The expressions of fear from the face admittedly belong to this category and may conceivably activate this region of the limbic system in a systematic way because they actually represent a prototypical instance of relevant signals in many situations.

Studies of emotion, particularly of fear processing, have recently burgeoned in the functional brain-imaging research. They have brought many valuable insights into the neurobiology of fear perception, but also more generally into the neural bases of face processing and conscious awareness. This rapidly growing literature has given support to the intuition that faces and facial expression are uniquely salient social stimuli, for which the human brain has dedicated and efficient processing capabilities. In addition, findings provided by functional brain-imaging techniques may offer new perspectives on the operations of highly specialized and "modular" systems in the brain, such as fear perception in the amygdala, and therefore also foster new concepts about the integration of such modular systems within distributed and interactive networks.

REFERENCES

Adolphs, R. (1999). Social cognition and the human brain. *Trends Cogn. Sci.* 3: 469-479.

Adolphs, R., Tranel, D., Damasio, H., and Damasio, A. (1994). Impaired recognition of emotion in facial expressions following bilateral damage to the human amygdala. *Nature* 372: 669-72.

Allison, T., Puce, A., and McCarthy, G. (2000). Social perception from visual cues: role of the STS region. *Trends Cogn. Sci.* 4: 267-278.

Amaral, D.G., Price, J.L., Pitkanen, A., and Carmichael, S.T. (1992). Anatomical organization of the primate amygdaloid complex. In: J. Aggleton (Ed.), The Amygdala: *Neurobiological Aspects of Emotion, Memory, And Mental Dysfunction.* New-York: Wiley-Liss, pp. 1-66.

Anderson, A.K., and Phelps, E.A. (2001). Lesions of the human amygdala impair enhanced perception of emotionally salient events. *Nature* 411: 305-9.

Armony, J.L., and LeDoux, J.E. (2000). How danger is encoded: Towards a systems, cellular, and computational understanding of cognitive-emotional interactions in fear. In: Gazzaniga MS, editor. *The New Cognitive Neurosciences.* Cambridge, MA: MIT Press, pp. 1067-1080.

Azzopardi, P., and Cowey, A. (1998). Blindsight and visual awareness. *Conscious Cogn.* 7: 292-311.

Bandettini, P.A. (1999). The temporal resolution of functional MRI. In: C.T.W. Moonen and P.A. Bandettini (eds.), *Functional MRI.* Berlin: Springer Verlag, pp. 205-220.

Baars, B. (1988). *A Cognitive theory of consciousness.* Cambridge, UK: Cambridge University Press.

Barbur JL, Watson JD, Frackowiak RS, and Zeki S. (1993). Conscious visual perception without V1. *Brain* 116: 1293-302.

Baylis, G., Rafal, R., and Driver, J. (1993). Visual extinction and stimulus repetition. *Journal of Cognitive Neuroscience* 5: 453-466.

Beale, J.M., and Keil, F.C. (1995). Categorical effects in the perception of faces. *Cognition* 57: 217-39.

Bechara, A., Tranel, D., Damasio, H., Adolphs, R., Rockland, C., and Damasio, A.R. (1995). Double dissociation of conditioning and declarative knowledge relative to the amygdala and hippocampus in humans. *Science* 269: 1115-8.

Benson, P. J. and Perrett, D. I. (1991). Synthesising continuous-tone caricatures. *Image and Vision Comput.* 9: 123-129.

Blair, R.J., Morris, J.S., Frith, C.D., Perrett, D.I., and Dolan, R.J. (1999). Dissociable neural responses to facial expressions of sadness and anger. *Brain* 122: 883-893.

Borod, J.C., Pick, L.H., Hall, S., Sliwinski, M., Madigan, N., Obler, L.K., Welkowitz, J., Canino, E., Erhan, H.M., Goral, M., Morrison, C., and Tabert, M. (2000). Relationships among facial, prosodic, and lexical channels of emotional perceptual processing. *Cognition and Emotion* 14: 193-211.

Breiter, H.C., Etcoff, N.L., Whalen, P.J., Kennedy, W.A., Rauch, S.L., Buckner, R.L., Strauss, M.M., Hyman, S.E., and Rosen, B.R. (1996). Response and habituation of the human amygdala during visual processing of facial expression. *Neuron* 17: 875-87.

Breitmeyer, B.G. (1984). *Visual Masking: an Integrative Approach.* Oxford: Clarendon.

Bruce, V., and Young, A.W. (1986). Understanding face recognition. *British Journal of Psychology* 77: 305-27.

Buchel, C., and Dolan, R.J. (2000). Classical fear conditioning in functional neuroimaging. *Curr. Opin. Neurobiol.* 10: 219-23.

Calder, A.J., Young, A.W., Keane, J., and Dean, M. (2000). Configural information in facial expression perception. *J. Exp. Psychol. Hum. Percept. Perform.* 26: 527-51.

Calder, A., Lawrence, A., and Young, A. (2001). Neuropsychology of fear and loathing. *Nat. Rev. Neurosci.* 2: 352-363.

Campanella, S., Quinet, P., Bruyer, R., Crommelinck, M., and Guerit, J.M. (2002). Categorical perception of happiness and fear facial expressions: an ERP study. *J. Cogn. Neurosci.* 14: 210-27.

Canli, T., Sivers, H., Whitfield, S.L., Gotlib, I.H., and Gabrieli, J.D. (2002). Amygdala response to happy faces as a function of extraversion. *Science* 296: 2191.

Clore, G.L., and Ortony, A. (2000). Cognition in emotion: always, sometimes or never? In: R. Lane and L. Nadel (eds.), *Cognitive neuroscience of emotions*. Oxford: Oxford University Press, pp. 24-61.

Coltheart, M. (1999). Modularity and cognition. *Trends in Cognitive Sciences* 3: 115-120.

Corbetta, M., and Shulman, G.L. (2002). Control of goal-directed and stimulus-driven attention in the brain. *Nat. Rev. Neurosci.* 3: 201-15.

Cordes, D., Turski, P.A., and Sorenson, J.A. (2000). Compensation of susceptibility-induced signal loss in echo-planar imaging for functional applications. *Magn. Reson. Imaging.* 18: 1055-68.

Cowey, A., and Stoerig, P. (1991). The neurobiology of blindsight. *Trends Neurosci.* 14: 140-5.

Critchley, H., Daly, E., Phillips, M., Brammer, M., Bullmore, E., Williams, S., Van Amelsvoort, T., Robertson, D., David, A., and Murphy, D. (2000). Explicit and implicit neural mechanisms for processing of social information from facial expressions: a functional magnetic resonance imaging study. *Hum. Brain Mapp.* 9: 93-105.

Critchley, H.D., Mathias, C.J., and Dolan, R.J. (2002). Fear conditioning in humans: the influence of awareness and autonomic arousal on functional neuroanatomy. *Neuron* 33: 653-63.

Damasio, A.R. (1994). Descartes'Error. *Emotion, Reason and the human brain.* New-York: Putnam Books.

Damasio, A.R. (1998). Emotion in the perspective of an integrated nervous system. *Brain Res. Rev.* 26: 83-6.

Damasio, A.R. (1999). The feeling of what happens. *Body and emotion in the making of consciousness.* New-York: Harcourt Brace and Company.

Darwin, C. (1872). The Expression of Emotions in Man and Animals. London: John Murray.

Davidson,. R.J., and Sutton, S.K. (1995). Affective neuroscience: the emergence of a discipline. *Curr. Opin. Neurobiol.* 5: 217-24.

de Gelder, B., Teunisse J.P., and Benson, P.J. (1997) Categorical perception of facial expressions: Categories and their internal structure. *Cognition and Emotion* 11: 1-23.

de Gelder, B., Vroomen, J., Pourtois, G. and Weiskrantz, L. (1999) Non-conscious recognition of affect in the absence of striate cortex. *Neuroreport* 10: 3759-63.

de Gelder, B., Pourtois, G., van Raamsdonk, M., Vroomen, J., and Weiskrantz, L. (2001). Unseen stimuli modulate conscious visual experience: evidence from inter-hemispheric summation. *Neuroreport* 12: 385-91.

de Gelder, B., Pourtois, G., and Weiskrantz, L. (2002). Fear recognition in the voice is modulated by unconsciously recognized facial expressions but not by unconsciously recognized affective pictures. *Proc. Natl. Acad. Sci. USA* 99: 4121-6.

D'Esposito, M., Zarahn, E., and Aguirre, G.K. (1999). Event-related functional MRI: implications for cognitive psychology. *Psychol. Bull.* 125: 155-64.

Dolan, R. J. (2000). Emotional processing in the human brain revealed through functional neuroimaging. In M. S. Gazzaniga (Ed.), *The new cognitive neurosciences* (2nd ed.). Cambridge, MA: MIT Press, pp. 1115-1131.

Dolan, R.J., and Morris, J.S. (2000). The functional anatomy of innate and acquired fear: perspectives from neuroimaging. In: Lane RD and Nadel L, editors. *Cognitive neuroscience of emotion.* New York: Oxford University Press, pp. 225-241.

Dolan, R.J., Morris, J.S., and de Gelder, B. (2001). Crossmodal binding of fear in voice and face. *Proc. Natl. Acad. Sci. USA* 98: 10006-10.

Drevets, W.C., and Raichle, M.E. (1998). Suppression of Regional Cerebral Blood during Emotional versus Higher Cognitive Implications for Interactions between Emotion and Cognition. *Cognition and Emotion* 12: 353-385.

Driver, J., and Mattingley, J.B. (1998). Parietal neglect and visual awareness. *Nat. Neurosci.* 1: 17-22.

Driver, J., and Vuilleumier, P. (2001). Perceptual awareness and its loss in unilateral neglect and extinction. *Cognition* 79: 39-88.

Ekman, P. (1992). An argument for basic emotions. *Cognition and Emotions* 6: 169-200.

Ekman, P., and Friesen, W.V. (1976). *Pictures of facial affect.* Palo-Alto: Consulting Psychologists Press.

Ekman, P., and Davidson, R.J. (1995). *The Nature of Emotion - Fundamental Questions.* Oxford: Oxford University Press.

Esteves, F., and Öhman, A. (1993). Masking the face: recognition of emotional facial expressions as a function of the parameters of backward masking. *Scand. J. Psychol.* 34: 1-18.

Eastwood, J. D., Smilek, D., and Merikle, P. M. (2001). Differential attentional guidance by unattended faces expressing positive and negative emotion. *Perception and Psychophysics* 63: 1004-1013.

Esteves, F., Parra, C., Dimberg, U., and Öhman, A. (1994). Nonconscious associative learning: Pavlovian conditioning of skin conductance responses to masked fear-relevant facial stimuli. *Psychophysiology* 31: 375-85.

Etcoff, N.L., and Magee, J.J. (1992). Categorical perception of facial expressions. *Cognition* 44: 227-40.

Fodor, J.A. (1983). *The Modularity of Mind. Cambridge,* MA: MIT Press.

Fox E. (2002). Processing emotional facial expressions: the role of anxiety and awareness. *Cogn. Affect. Behav. Neurosci.* 2: 52-63.

Frijda, N. (1989). *The emotions.* Cambridge: CUP.

Friston, K.J., Frith, C.D., Liddle, P.F., and Frackowiak, R.S. (1993). Functional connectivity: the principal-component analysis of large (PET) data sets. *J. Cereb. Blood Flow Metab.* 13: 5-14.

Fuster, J.M. (2000). The module: Crisis of a paradigm. *Neuron.* 26: 51-53.

George, N., Driver, J., and Dolan, R.J. (2001). Seen gaze-direction modulates fusiform activity and its coupling with other brain areas during face processing. *Neuroimage* 13: 1102-12.

Golby, A.J., Gabrieli, J.D., Chiao, J.Y., and Eberhardt, J.L. (2001). Differential responses in the fusiform region to same-race and other-race faces. *Nat. Neurosci.* 4: 845-50.

Gorno-Tempini, M.L., Pradelli, S., Serafini, M., Pagnoni, G., Baraldi, P., Porro, C., Nicoletti, R., Umita, C., and Nichelli, P. (2001). Explicit and incidental facial expression processing: an fMRI study. *Neuroimage* 14: 465-73.

Halgren, E., Babb, T.L., and Crandall, P.H. (1978). Activity of human hippocampal formation and amygdala neurons during memory testing. *Electroencephalogr. Clin. Neurophysiol.* 45: 585-601.

Hamann, S.B., Ely, T.D., Hoffman, J.M., and Kilts, C.D. (2002). Ecstasy and agony: activation of the human amygdala in positive and negative emotion. *Psychol. Sci.* 13: 135-41.

Hamm, A.O., Weike, A.I., Schupp, H.T., Treig, T., Dressel, A., and Kessler, C. (2003). Affective blindsight: intact fear conditioning to a visual cue in a cortically blind patient. *Brain* 126: 267-75.

Hansen, C. H., and Hansen, R. D. (1988). Finding the face in the crowd: An anger superiority effect. *Journal of Personality and Social Psychology* 54: 917-924.

Hariri, A.R., Bookheimer, S.Y., and Mazziotta, J.C. (2000). Modulating emotional responses: effects of a neocortical network on the limbic system. *Neuroreport* 11: 43-8.

Hariri, A.R., Tessitore, A., Mattay, V.S., Fera, F., and Weinberger, D.R. (2002). The amygdala response to emotional stimuli: a comparison of faces and scenes. *Neuroimage* 17: 317-23.

Hariri, A.R., Mattay, V.S., Tessitore, A., Kolachana, B., Fera, F., Goldman, D., Egan, M.F., and Weinberger, D.R. (2002). Serotonin transporter genetic variation and the response of the human amygdala. *Science* 297: 400-3.

Harnad, S. (1987). Categorical perception: *The groundwork of cognition.* Cambridge, MA: CUP.

Haxby, J.V., Ishai, A., Chao, L.L., Ungerleider, L.G., and Martin A. (2000). Object-form topology in the ventral temporal lobe: Response to I. Gauthier (2000). *Trends Cogn. Sci.* 4: 3-4.

Haxby, J.V., Gobbini, M.I., Furey, M.L., Ishai, A., Schouten, J.L., and Pietrini, P. (2001). Distributed and overlapping representations of faces and objects in ventral temporal cortex. *Science* 293: 2425-30.

Irwin, W., Davidson, R.J., Lowe, M.J., Mock, B.J., Sorenson, J.A., and Turski, P.A. (1996). Human amygdala activation detected with echo-planar functional magnetic resonance imaging. *Neuroreport* 7: 1765-9.

Kahn, I., Yeshurun, Y., Rotshtein, P., Fried, I., Ben-Bashat, D., and Hendler, T. (2002). The role of the amygdala in signaling prospective outcome of choice. *Neuron.*33: 983-94.

Kanwisher, N. (2000). Domain specificity in face perception. *Nat. Neurosci.* 3: 759-63.

Kanwisher, N., McDermott, J., and Chun, M.M. (1997). The fusiform face area: a module in human extrastriate cortex specialized for face perception. *J. Neurosci.* 17: 4302-11.

Karnath, H.O., Ferber, S., and Himmelbach, M. (2001). Spatial awareness is a function of the temporal not the posterior parietal lobe. *Nature* 411: 950-3.

Kastner, S., Pinsk, M.A., De Weerd, P., Desimone, R., and Ungerleider, L.G. (1999). Increased activity in human visual cortex during directed attention in the absence of visual stimulation. *Neuron* 22: 751-61.

Kastner, S., and Ungerleider, L.G. (2000). Mechanisms of visual attention in the human cortex. *Annu. Rev. Neurosci.* 23: 315-41.

Kawashima, R., Sugiura, M., Kato, T., Nakamura, A., Hatano, K., Ito, K., Fukuda, H., Kojima, S., and Nakamura, K. (1999). The human amygdala plays an important role in gaze monitoring. A PET study. *Brain* 122: 779-83.

Keightley, M.L., Grady, C.L., Graham, S., Winocur, G., and Mayberg, H.S. (2000). Separate brain systems for emotional processing of faces and pictures. *Abstract Soc. Neurosci.* 755.16.

Kentridge, R.W., Heywood, C.A., and Weiskrantz, L. (1999). Attention without awareness in blindsight. *Proc. R. Soc. Lond. B. Biol. Sci.* 266: 1805-11.

Kim, S.-G., Lee, S.P., Goodyear, B., and Silva, A.C. (1999). Spatial resolution of BOLD and other fMRI techniques. In: C.T.W. Moonen and P.A. Bandettini (eds.), *Functional MRI.* Berlin: Springer Verlag, pp. 195-203.

Klüver, H., and Bucy, P.C. (1938). An analysis of functions of the temporal lobes in monkeys, with special reference to "psychic blindness". *J. Psychol.* 5: 33-54.

Kohler, S., and Moscovitch M. (1997). Unconscious visual processing in neuropsychological syndromes: a survey of the literature and evaluation of models of cousciousness. In: M.D. Rugg (Ed.) *Cognitive Neuroscience.* Cambridge, Massachusetts: The MIT Press, pp. 305-372.

Kolb, B., and Taylor, L. (2000). Facial expression, emotion, and hemispheric organisation. In: R. Lane and L. Nadel (eds.), *Cognitive neuroscience of emotions.* Oxford: Oxford University Press, pp. 62-83.

LaBar, K.S., LeDoux, J.E., Spencer, D.D., and Phelps, E.A. (1995). Impaired fear conditioning following unilateral temporal lobectomy in humans. *J. Neurosci.* 15: 6846-55.

LaBar, K.S., Gatenby, J.C., Gore, J.C., LeDoux, J.E., and Phelps, E.A. (1998). Human amygdala activation during conditioned fear acquisition and extinction: a mixed-trial fMRI study. *Neuron* 20: 937-45.

LaBar, K.S., Gitelman, D.R., Mesulam, M.M., and Parrish, T.B. (2001a). Impact of signal-to-noise on functional MRI of the human amygdala. *Neuroreport* 12: 3461-4.

LaBar, K.S., Gitelman, D.R., Parrish, T.B., Kim, Y.H., Nobre, A.C., and Mesulam, M.M. (2001b). Hunger selectively modulates corticolimbic activation to food stimuli in humans. *Behav. Neurosci.* 115: 493-500.

Lamme, V.A. (2001). Blindsight: the role of feedforward and feedback corticocortical connections. *Acta Psychol.* (Amst) 107: 209-28.

Lane, R.D., Reiman, E.M., Ahern, G.L., Schwartz, G.E., and Davidson, R.J. (1997). Neuroanatomical correlates of happiness, sadness, and disgust. *Am. J. Psychiatry.* 154: 926-33.

Lane, R.D., Reiman, E.M., Axelrod, B., Yun, L.S., Holmes, A., and Schwartz, G.E. (1998). Neural correlates of levels of emotional awareness. Evidence of an interaction between emotion and attention in the anterior cingulate cortex. *J. Cogn. Neurosci.* 10: 525-35.

Lane, R.D., and Nadel, L. (2000). *Cognitive neuroscience of emotion.* New York: Oxford University Press.

Lang, P.J., Bradley, M.M. and Cuthbert, B.N. (1995). The International Affective Picture System (IAPS): Photographic slides. Gainesville: *The Center for Research in Psychophysiology.*

Lavie, N. (1995). Perceptual load as a necessary condition for selective attention. *J. Exp. Psychol. Hum. Percept. Perform.* 21: 451-68.

Lazarus, R.S. (1984). On the primacy of cognition. *American Psychologist.* 39: 124-129.

LeDoux, J. (1996). *The emotional brain: the mysterious underpinnings of emotional life.* New-York: Simon and Schuster.

Leonard, C.M., Rolls, E.T., Wilson, F.A., and Baylis, G.C. (1985). Neurons in the amygdala of the monkey with responses selective for faces. *Behav. Brain Res.* 15: 159-76.

Logothetis, N.K., Pauls, J., Augath, M., Trinath, T., and Oeltermann, A. (2001). Neurophysiological investigation of the basis of the fMRI signal. *Nature* 412: 150-7.

Macknik, S.L., and Livingstone, M.S. (1998). Neuronal correlates of visibility and invisibility in the primate visual system. *Nat. Neurosci.* 1: 144-9.

McKelvie, S.J. (1995). Emotional expression in upside-down faces: evidence for configurational and componential processing. *British Journal of Social Psychology* 34: 325-34.

Merboldt, K.D., Fransson, P., Bruhn, H., and Frahm, J. (2001). Functional MRI of the human amygdala? *Neuroimage* 14: 253-7.

Mogg, K., McNamara, J., Powys, M., Rawlinson, H., Seiffer, A., and Bradley, B.P. (2000). Selective attention to threat: A test of two cognitive models of anxiety. *Cognition and Emotion* 14: 375-399.

Morris, J.S., Frith, C.D., Perrett, D.I., Rowland, D., Young, A.W., Calder, A.J., and Dolan, R.J. (1996). A differential neural response in the human amygdala to fearful and happy facial expressions. *Nature* 383: 812-5.

Morris, J.S., Öhman, A., and Dolan, R.J. (1998a). Conscious and unconscious emotional learning in the human amygdala. *Nature* 393: 467-70.

Morris, J.S., Friston, K.J., Buchel, C., Frith, C.D., Young, A.W., Calder, A.J., and Dolan, R.J. (1998b). A neuromodulatory role for the human amygdala in processing emotional facial expressions. *Brain* 121: 47-57.

Morris, J.S., Öhman, A., and Dolan, R.J. (1999). A subcortical pathway to the right amygdala mediating "unseen" fear. *Proc. Natl. Acad. Sci. U S A* 96: 1680-5.

Morris, J.S., Buchel, C., and Dolan, R.J. (2001a). Parallel neural responses in amygdala subregions and sensory cortex during implicit fear conditioning. *Neuroimage* 13: 1044-52.

Morris, J.S., de Gelder, B., Weiskrantz, L., and Dolan, R.J. (2001b). Differential extrageniculostriate and amygdala responses to presentation of emotional faces in a cortically blind field. *Brain* 124: 1241-52.

Morris, J.S., deBonis, M., and Dolan, R.J. (2002). Human amygdala responses to fearful eyes. *Neuroimage* 17: 214-22.

Narumoto, J., Okada, T., Sadato, N., Fukui, K., and Yonekura, Y. (2001). Attention to emotion modulates fMRI activity in human right superior temporal sulcus. *Brain Res. Cogn. Brain Res.* 12: 225-31.

Nelson, C.A., and Dolgin, K. (1985). The generalized discrimination of facial expressions by seven-month-old infants. *Child Development* 56: 58-61.

Nelson, C.A., Morse, D.A., and Leavitt, L.A. (1979). Recognition of facial expressions by seven-month-old infants. *Child Development* 50: 1239-42.

Öhman, A. (1986). Face the beast and fear the face: animal and social fears as prototypes for evolutionary analyses of emotion. *Psychophysiology* 23: 123-45.

Öhman, A., Flykt, A., and Lundqvist, D. (2000). Unconscious emotion: evolutionary perspectives, psychophysiological data and neuropsychological mechanisms. In: R. Lane and L. Nadel (eds.), *Cognitive neuroscience of emotions*. Oxford: Oxford University Press, pp. 296-327.

Öhman, A., Lundqvist, D., and Esteves, F. (2001). The face in the crowd revisited: a threat advantage with schematic stimuli. *J. Pers. Soc. Psychol.* 80: 381-96.

Öhman, A., and Mineka, S. (2001). Fears, phobias, and preparedness: toward an evolved module of fear and fear learning. *Psychol. Rev.* 108: 483-522.

Olshausen, B.A., Anderson, C.H,, and Van Essen, D.C. (1993). A neurobiological model of visual attention and invariant pattern recognition based on dynamic routing of information. *J. Neurosci.* 13: 4700-19.

Panksepp, J. (1998). Affective Neuroscience: *The Foundations of Human and Animal Emotions*. New-York: Oxford University Press.

Pavlov, I. (1927). *Conditioned reflexes*. New York: Dover.

Perrett, D.I., Hietanen, J.K., Oram, M.W., and Benson, P.J. (1992). Organization and functions of cells responsive to faces in the temporal cortex. *Philos. Trans. R. Soc. Lond. B. Biol. Sci.* 335: 23-30.

Perrett, D.I., May, K.A., and Yoshikawa, S. (1994). Facial shape and judgements of female attractiveness. *Nature* 368: 239-42.

Pessoa, L., McKenna, M., Gutierrez, E., and Ungerleider, L.G. (2002). Neural processing of emotional faces requires attention. *Proc. Natl. Acad. Sci. U S A* 99: 11458-63.

Phelps, E.A. (2001). Faces and races in the brain. *Nat. Neurosci.* 4: 775-6.

Phelps, E.A., O'Connor, K.J., Cunningham, W.A., Funayama, E.S., Gatenby, J.C., Gore, J.C., and Banaji, M.R. (2000). Performance on indirect measures of race evaluation predicts amygdala activation. *J. Cogn. Neurosci.* 12: 729-38.

Phelps, E.A., O'Connor, K.J., Gatenby, J.C., Gore, J.C., Grillon, C., and Davis, M. (2001). Activation of the left amygdala to a cognitive representation of fear. *Nat. Neurosci.* 4: 437-41.

Phillips, M.L., Young, A.W., Senior, C., Brammer, M., Andrew, C., Calder, A.J., Bullmore, E.T., Perrett, D.I., Rowland, D., Williams, S.C., Gray, J.A., and David, A.S. (1997). A specific neural substrate for perceiving facial expressions of disgust. *Nature* 389: 495-8.

Phillips, M.L., Medford, N., Young, A.W., Williams, L., Williams, S.C., Bullmore, E.T., Gray, J.A., and Brammer, M.J. (2001). Time courses of left and right amygdalar responses to fearful facial expressions. *Hum. Brain Mapp.* 12: 193-202.

Poppel, E., Held, R., and Frost, D. (1973). Residual visual function after brain wounds involving the central visual pathways in man. *Nature* 243: 295-6.

Posner, M. I. (1978) *Chronometric explorations of mind.* Erlbaum.

Posner, M. I., Walker, J. A., Friedrich, F. J., and Rafal, R. (1984). Effects of parietal injury on covert orienting of visual attention. *Journal of Neuroscience* 4: 1863-1874.

Posner, M.I., Petersen, S.E., Fox, P.T., and Raichle, M.E. (1988). Localization of cognitive operations in the human brain. *Science* 240: 1627-31.

Posner, M.I., and Raichle, M.E. (1997). *Images of Mind.* Scientific American Library, New York.

Raichle, M.E. (2001). Bold insights. *Nature* 412: 128-30.

Rauch, S.L., Whalen, P.J., Shin, L.M., McInerney, S.C., Macklin, M.L., Lasko, N.B., Orr, S.P., and Pitman, R.K. (2000). Exaggerated amygdala response to masked facial stimuli in posttraumatic stress disorder: a functional MRI study. *Biol. Psychiatry* 47: 769-76.

Rolls, E.T. (1999). *The brain and emotion.* Oxford: Oxford University Press.

Rosenkranz, J.A., and Grace, A.A. (2002). Dopamine-mediated modulation of odour-evoked amygdala potentials during pavlovian conditioning. *Nature* 417: 282-7.

Savoy, R.L. (2001). History and future directions of human brain mapping and functional neuroimaging. *Acta Psychologica* 107: 9-42.

Schwartz, C.E., Wright, C.I., Shin, L.M., Kagan, J., and Rauch, S.L. (2003). Inhibited and uninhibited infants "grown up": adult amygdalar response to novelty. *Science* 300: 1952-3.

Spiridon, M., and Kanwisher, N. (2002). How distributed is visual category information in human occipito-temporal cortex? An fMRI study. *Neuron* 35: 1157-65.

Sprengelmeyer, R., Rausch, M., Eysel, U.T., and Przuntek, H. (1998). Neural structures associated with recognition of facial expressions of basic emotions. *Proc. R. Soc. Lond. B. Biol. Sci.* 265: 1927-31.

Sugase, Y., Yamane, S., Ueno, S., and Kawano, K. (1999). Global and fine information coded by single neurons in the temporal visual cortex. *Nature* 400: 869-73.

Tabert, M.H., Borod, J.C., Tang, C.Y., Lange, G., Wei, T.C., Johnson, R., Nusbaum, A.O., and Buchsbaum, M.S. (2001). Differential amygdala activation during emotional decision and recognition memory tasks using unpleasant words: an fMRI study. *Neuropsychologia* 39: 556-73.

Talairach, J., and Tournoux, P. (1988). *Co-Planar Stereotaxic Atlas of the Human Brain.* New York: Thieme Medical Publishers Inc.

Tarr, M.J., and Gauthier, I. (2000). FFA: a flexible fusiform area for subordinate-level visual processing automatized by expertise. *Nat. Neurosci.* 3: 764-9.

Taylor, S.F., Liberzon, I., Fig, L.M., Decker, L.R., Minoshima, S., and Koeppe, R.A. (1998). The effect of emotional content on visual recognition memory: a PET activation study. *Neuroimage* 8: 188-97.

Tong, F. (2003). Primary visual cortex and visual awareness. *Nat. Rev. Neurosci.* 4: 219-29.

Treisman, A.M., and Gelade, G. (1980). A feature-integration theory of attention. *Cognit. Psychol.* 12: 97-136.

Vallar, G. (1993). The anatomical basis of spatial neglect in humans. In: Robertson IH and Marshall J, eds. *Unilateral Neglect: Clinical and Experimental Studies.* Hove: Lawrence Erlbaum Associates, pp. 27-53.

Vuilleumier, P. (2002). Facial expression and selective attention. *Current Opinion in Psychiatry* 15: 291-300.

Vuilleumier, P., Armony, J.L., Driver, J., and Dolan, R.J. (2001a). Effects of attention and emotion on face processing in the human brain: an event-related fMRI study. *Neuron* 30: 829-41.

Vuilleumier, P., Sagiv, N., Hazeltine, E., Poldrack, R.A., Swick, D., Rafal, R.D., and Gabrieli, J.D. (2001b). Neural fate of seen and unseen faces in visuospatial neglect: a combined event-related functional MRI and event-related potential study. *Proc. Natl. Acad. Sci. U S A* 98: 3495-500.

Vuilleumier, P., and Schwartz, S. (2001a). Emotional facial expressions capture attention. *Neurology* 56: 153-8.

Vuilleumier, P., and Schwartz, S. (2001b). Beware and be aware: capture of spatial attention by fear-related stimuli in neglect. *Neuroreport* 12: 1119-22.

Vuilleumier, P., Armony, J.L., Clarke, K., Husain, M., Driver, J., and Dolan, R.J. (2002). Neural response to emotional faces with and without awareness: event-related fMRI in a parietal patient with visual extinction and spatial neglect. *Neuropsychologia* 40: 2156-66.

Vuilleumier, P., Armony, J.L., Driver, J., and Dolan, R.J. (2003). Distinct spatial frequency sensitivities for processing faces and emotional expressions. *Nat. Neurosci.* 6: 624-31.

Vuilleumier, P., Armony, J.L., and Dolan, R.J. (2004). Reciprocal links between emotion and attention. In: RJS Frackowiak and J Mazziotta (Eds). *Human Brain Mapping.* London: Elsevier, pp. 419-444

Weiskrantz, L. (1956). Behavioral changes associated with ablation of the amygdaloid complex in monkeys. *J. Comp. Psychol.* 49: 381-391.

Weiskrantz, L. (1986). Blindsight. *A case study and implications.* Oxford: Oxford University Press.

Weiskrantz, L. (1997). *Consciousness Lost and Found.* Oxford: Oxford University Press.

Weiskrantz, L. (2000). Blindsight: implications for the conscious experience of emotion. In: R. Lane, and L. Nadel (Eds.) *Cognitive neuroscience of emotions.* Oxford: Oxford University Press, pp. 277-295.

Weiskrantz, L., Warrington, E.K., Sanders, M.D., and Marshall, J. (1974). Visual capacity in the hemianopic field following a restricted occipital ablation. *Brain* 97: 709-28.

Whalen, P.J., Rauch, S.L., Etcoff, N.L., McInerney, S.C., Lee, M.B., and Jenike, M.A. (1998). Masked presentations of emotional facial expressions modulate amygdala activity without explicit knowledge. *J. Neurosci.* 18: 411-8.

Whalen, P.J., Shin, L.M., McInerney, S.C., Fischer, H., Wright, C.I., and Rauch, S.L. (2001). A functional MRI study of human amygdala responses to facial expressions of fear versus anger. *Emotion* 1: 70-83.

Williams, L.M., Phillips, M.L., Brammer, M.J., Skerrett, D., Lagopoulos, J., Rennie, C., Bahramali, H., Olivieri, G., David, A.S., Peduto, A., and Gordon, E. (2001). Arousal dissociates amygdala and hippocampal fear responses: evidence from simultaneous fMRI and skin conductance recording. *Neuroimage* 14: 1070-9.

Winston, J.S., Strange, B.A., O'Doherty, J., and Dolan, R.J. (2002). Automatic and intentional brain responses during evaluation of trustworthiness of faces. *Nat. Neurosci.* 5: 277-83.

Wojciulik, E., Kanwisher, N., and Driver, J. (1998). Covert visual attention modulates face-specific activity in the human fusiform gyrus: fMRI study. *J. Neurophysiol.* 79: 1574-8.

Wright, C.I., Fischer, H., Whalen, P.J., McInerney, S.C., Shin, L.M., and Rauch, S.L. (2001). Differential prefrontal cortex and amygdala habituation to repeatedly presented emotional stimuli. *Neuroreport* 12: 379-83.

Wright, C.I., Martis, B., Schwartz, C.E., Shin, L.M., Fischer, H.H., McMullin, K., and Rauch, S.L. (2003). Novelty responses and differential effects of order in the amygdala, substantia innominata, and inferior temporal cortex. *Neuroimage* 18: 660-9.

Yamasaki, H., LaBar, K.S., and McCarthy, G. (2002). Dissociable prefrontal brain systems for attention and emotion. *Proc. Natl. Acad. Sci. U S A* 99: 11447-51.

Young, A.W., Hellawell, D., and Hay, D.C. (1987). Configurational information in face perception. *Perception* 16: 747-59.

Young, A.W., Rowland, D., Calder, A.J., Etcoff, N.L., Seth, A., and Perrett, D.I. (1997). Facial expression megamix: tests of dimensional and category accounts of emotion recognition. *Cognition* 63: 271-313.

Zajonc, R.B. (1980). Feeling and thinking – preferences need no inferences. *American Psychologist* 35: 151-175.

Zald, D.H. (2003). The human amygdala and the emotional evaluation of sensory stimuli. *Brain Res. Rev.* 41: 88-123.

In: Fear in Cognitive Neuroscience
Editor: Salvatore Campanella, pp. 97-115
ISBN: 1-59454-502-2

Chapter 5

EMOTIONS AND FEAR: FROM NEUROBIOLOGICAL MECHANISMS TO PHARMACOLOGICAL INTERVENTIONS

Emmanuel Streel[1], Valérie Antoniali[1], Mike Kyrios[2], Isy Pelc[1] and Paul Verbanck[1]

[1] Université Libre de Bruxelles - CHU Brugmann – Service de Psychiatrie - Laboratoire de Psychologie Médicale Alcoologie et Toxicomanies - Unité de recherche sur la Biologie des dépendances - Brussels – Belgium

[2] University of Melbourne – Departments of Psychology and Psychiatry – Parkville – Victoria - Australia

INTRODUCTION

In their fascinating book published in 1911, " les manifestations fonctionnelles des Psychonévroses, leur traitement par la psychothérapie ", Dejerine and Gaukler highlighted the part emotions play in various clinical manifestations. This fact is not new in itself, however, contrary to what one could expect, the authors do not limit themselves to the implication of emotions on the genesis of "psychoneuroses", a very common thing at that time, but they largely exceed this reductionistic framework and develop the part that emotions can play on somatic perturbations. The authors specify, as an example, that digestive, cardiac or respiratory disorders, motor or sensitive inhibitions, vasomotor or secretary actions, can be created by negative emotions directly or after a period of rumination (Dejerine and Gauckler, 1911). The authors describe anguish in a very precise way and describe it as a physical diffusion of a psychic emotion which gradually develops in the consciousness and which psychically creates anxiety on which anguish is often dependent. We will not enter in the historical debate of dissociating anguish and anxiety here, but we can however note how much the authors consider the emotions as a sort of psychic/physic interface. Although one might consider that early conceptualisations of emotion were rudimentary in terms of "neurosciences", various authors already had a very clear notion that the body is mainly responsible for certain "complex nervous phenomena" of which emotions, including fear, are a part. In a synthesis of his work, Pavlov (1904) presents various experiments on conditioning and "reflexes". He develops the concept of "reflexes" and specifies two aspects that refer to the functions of higher structures of animal nervous systems. On one hand, because reflexes represent one of the most complex phenomena in human behaviour, they must necessarily be related to higher stages of the nervous system. On the other hand, based on animal experiments following total or partial hemispheric removal, it was evident that reflexes require the intervention of the cerebral hemispheres. Interestingly, Pavlov (1904) noted that following extirpation of specific brain areas, animals became "softer" or "more aggressive", although he was critical of experiments that failed to define these concepts before associating them with particular cerebral areas. From Darwin (1872) to LeDoux (2000), through Frijda (1989), Mac Lean (1949), Ekman (1992), Damasio (1994) and so many others, decades of research in the field of emotions has seen an important accumulation of knowledge and the development of theories of emotion. Such theories of emotion are in constant evolution, and today a growing number of researchers are focusing on the neurobiology of emotions in general and fear in particular. As pointed out by Kreek et al. (2002), technological advances in neurochemical techniques, molecular-biology approaches, behavioural-studies, coupled with an increasing interest in developing more appropriate animal models, have greatly increased our knowledge. Even if the concept of an "emotional brain" is still present in various publications, we notice the progressive growth of studies focusing on the neurochemistry of emotions. Even if the idea of molecules of emotions are considered as outrageous by certain (Pert, 1997), basic neurosciences and animal studies are carrying promising results in the identification of underlying mechanisms of emotions and, possibly leading to more efficient pharmacological interventions where pathology is present (e.g. Panic attack). In addition, psychological theories, such as cognitive-behavioural and information processing models, have also increased our knowledge of mental and other processes underlying emotional disorders (Eysenck, 1992), and are now informing neuroscientist research about important phenomenological aspects of such disorders.

In this chapter, we will take the reader from the emotional brain through the neurochemistry and both the pharmacological and psychological modulation of emotions. We will indicate for example the capacity of opioïds-peptides and related system (e.g. cannabinoids) in the interference of emotions and fear and also highlight the relationship between exogenous opioïds, cannabinoids, and mood perturbations. We will put before the reader information about pharmacological and psychological interventions and indicate potential new approaches in the management of the pathology where emotions and /or fear are mainly present.

Emotions: From Cerebral Localizations to Neuropeptides

An Emotional Brain?

What one is used to call the "emotional brain" refers conceptually to the limbic system. The concept of limbic system, limbic functions, and limbic structures, has exerted a considerable influence in neurosciences as well as its application in clinical practice (Kotter and Meyer, 1992). At the macroscopic level, the limbic system includes the cingulate gyrus, hippocampus, parahippocampal gyrus, amygdala, septal nuclei, and parts of the thalamus and hypothalamus (Le Doux, 2000). In addition, some of these structures encompass other concepts and structures such as the rhinencephalon, papez network, visceral brain, etc... (Kötter and Meyer, 1992). Today, although most scientists do not consider the brain as containing a distinct "emotional center" or that emotions are confined in specific localizations, the scientific data, however, agree on the important role that various structures play on emotions. In an article published in 1878, the neurologist Paul Broca indicated the presence, in all mammals, of a whole segment of cortical areas distinct from the surrounding cortex. Using the term "limbus" (Latin: limit), Broca named this segment of cortical areas forming an edge around the cerebral trunk, the limbic lobe (Bear et al., 1997). Around the 1930s, certain limbic structures were discovered to play a part in the emotional processes, in particular via the works of Papez. Papez proposed that the emotional process was related to the activity of various cerebral areas, in particular the cingular cortex. Later on, the limbic system was integrated in the context of an evolutionary explanation of mind and behaviour (Mc Lean, 1949, 1952). Thinking, reasoning, learning and other cognitive process, were associated with the neocortex. In contrast, the old cortex and related subcortical areas from the limbic system, were associated to more rudimentary aspects of functioning, particularly, our emotions (LeDoux, 2000). The limbic system concept underwent severe criticism when it was discovered that damage to the hippocampus, the center piece of the limbic system, led to severe cognitive deficits (Scoville and Milner, 1957). This was incompatible with the original idea that the limbic system and its primitive architecture was poorly suited to cognitive functions (MacLean, 1949; 1952). Several attempts were made to reconsider the concept of the limbic system itself (e.g. Isaacson, 1982), with some authors recommending its total abandonment (LeDoux, 1991; Kötter and Meyer, 1992). Nevertheless, the concept of the limbic system survived, as much evidence supported its involvement in emotion, although there is little understanding of how our emotions could be the product of the limbic system (LeDoux, 1991). While the current scientific zeitgeist which focuses on localising various human functions to particular brain areas may be seen as a "new phrenology", animal studies may be less inclined to be criticised as they tend to examine cellular mechanisms (Blanchard et al., 2001).

Fear: From Fear-Conditioning to Neuropeptides

The stimuli of fear can be divided in two distinct categories: learned and unlearned. Unlearned stimuli evoke fear responses in animals at first exposure; in contrast, stimuli that do not initially evoke fear, do so after the animal has come to associate them with fear (Coupland, 2000). The fear conditioning paradigm on animals (mainly rats) has been extensively used in various experimental design. Using conditioning, fear has been considered as a set of processing circuits that detect and respond to aversive stimuli. Through this approach, fear was made experimentally tractable (LeDoux, 1991). Classical fear conditioning is an associative learning process in which subjects come to express fear responses to a neutral conditioned stimulus paired with an aversive unconditioned stimulus (Blair et al., 2001). Conditioned fear is mediated by the transmission of information about the conditioned stimulus and unconditioned stimulus to the amygdala, and the control of fear reactions via the amygdala outputs to behavioural, autonomic and endocrine control systems located in the brainstem (LeDoux, 2000). Longer-term adaptations suppose the development of more complex behavioural and cognitive responses mediated by the hippocampus, mediodorsal thalamus, prefrontal cortex and ventral striatum (Coupland, 2000). The activation of such a defence system also triggers the monoaminergic and cholinergic systems. The amygdala plays an essential role in the expression of fear conditioning (Davis, 1994; LeDoux, 1994), more precisely, the basolateral amygdala, including lateral, basolateral and basomedial nuclei (LeDoux, 2000; Maren, 1998). Numerous researches highlighted that both the acquisition and expression of conditioned fear requires neurons in the basolateral amygdala (Maren, 1999; Lee et al., 1996; Cousens and Otto, 1998). For example, neurotoxic lesions in the basolateral amygdala produce deficits in the acquisition and expression of conditioned responses to fear (e.g. freezing) (Maren et al., 1996). It has also been demonstrated that, as suggested by others (Kim and Davies, 1993), overtraining does not limit the important role of the basolateral amygdala in the acquisition and expression of fear conditioning (Maren, 1998). Fear conditioning has emerged as a leading paradigm for studying cellular mechanisms underlying learning and memory (Tang et al., 2003).

Amygdala lesion studies helped to identify the circuitry underlying fear conditioning, and questions slowly turned to the physiological plasticityÑ□elated to fear conditioning. Let us note that in parallel to this scientific passion for the amygdala, it is still unclear to what extent the association between conditioned and unconditioned stimuli are formed and stored within the basolateral amygdala (Tang et al., 2003). Some authors (Vazdarjanova and McGaugh, 1998; McGaugh, 2000; Cahill et al., 1999) suggest that an intact basolateral amygdala complex did not appear to be essential for the formation and expression of long-term cognitive/explicit memory of contextual fear conditioning. They consider that the amygdala could modulate memories that are formed elsewhere. However, as pointed out by others (Fanselow and LeDoux, 1999), evidence for the amygdala's role in modulation should not be confused with evidence against its role in plasticity. Nevertheless, even if several uncertainties remain to be explored, it has been demonstrated that the lateral nuclei seemed to be both the initial point of sensory processing and the initial site of plasticity in the amygdala (LeDoux, 2000; Quirk et al., 1995; 1997), and that long term potentiation, believed to engage cellular mechanisms similar to those underlying natural learning (Lynch, 1986), occurs in this fear processing pathway. Furthemore, the processing of natural stimuli similar to those used as conditioned stimuli is also facilitated the following of long term potentiation. Due to NMDA receptors being crucial for long term potentiation and long term depression (two forms of synaptic plasticity with information storage potential), it has been postulated that NMDA receptor-dependent synaptic plasticity in the amygdala is involved in fear conditioning (Hongjoo and Jeansok, 1998; Miserendino et al., 1990; LeDoux, 1993). Other authors also suggest that consolidation of the conditioned and unconditioned stimuli requires protein biosynthesis, activation of kinases and NMDA receptors (Tang et al., 2003). Several lines of evidence implies other mechanisms in the control of the neural substrates that command defensive behaviours (Eichenberger et al., 2002). These mechanisms implicate GABAergic, serotoninergic and opioïd- mediated mechanisms (Coimbra and Brandao, 1993; 1997; Cardoso et al., 1992; Schmitt et al., 1986). It having been established that the brain aversive system, (Graeff, 1990) including the medial hippothalamus, amygdala and mesencephalic structures, constitute the main neural substrates for aversive state integration in the brain. Eichenberger et al. (2002) examined the effects of central administration of two opioïd antagonists (naloxone and naltrexone) on the aversive response elicited by electrical and chemical stimulation of different mesencephalic structures. Their results showed that electrical and chemical (using bicuculline, a GABAa antagonist) stimulation of the midbrain tectum induced alertness, freezing and vigorous escape behaviours. Of particular interest, pre-treatment with central micro injection of opioïd antagonists (5 µg) 10 mins before chemical stimulation (of aversive sites located in the dorsal periaqueductal grey matter) caused a significant decrease in the fear-related responses induced. The potential interactions between opioïd peptides or serotonin and GABA (Tao and Auerbach, 2000) highlight the potential integrative circuitry (Eichenberger et al., 2002), including molecular and cellular underlying mechanisms, in the elaboration of fear and fear-induced analgesia in the central nervous system.

For many years, researchers have believed that emotions were controlled by certain parts of the brain; this "neurocentric" assumption was pertinent, but incomplete (Pert, 1997). We now agree that brain functions and behaviour are associated with neurobiological activity and a growing number of researches fuel the conviction in the concept of "molecules" of emotions (Pert, 1997). Researches indicate that peptides (e.g. opioïds) could constitute a good candidate as molecules of emotions. For example, identical opiate receptors could be found in the brain of all vertebrates. Even insects and other invertebrates have opiate receptors. Furthermore, brain limbic structures, involved in emotions, have been found to contain 85% to 95 % of various peptides (Pert, 1997). The discovery during the 1980s of numerous novel peptides in the central nervous system, each capable of regulating some aspect of a neural function, produced considerable excitement (Bloom, 2001). Although thought for a long time to be restricted to endocrine glands, peptides have been identified in various brain areas and seen to act with other categories of transmitters. Peptides can be organised by families (ancestral or concurrent) of anatomic patterns, as peptides follow consistent anatomical organisations or functions. In the field of the neurochemistry of emotions, one system which has attracted considerable attention involves a corticotrophin-releasing factor (CRF). This 41-amino acid peptide is hypothesized to play a role in coordinating endocrine functions as well as behavioural responses to stress (Takahashi, 2001; Radulovic et al., 1999). As fear and anxiety are common emotions related to stress, CRF has been considered to play an essential role in mediating these emotions. CRF and urocortin (a CRF-like peptide) act via two G protein-coupled receptor subtypes known as CRF1 (Chang et al., 1993) and CRF2 (Lovenberg et al., 1995). Targeted receptor alterations were used in order to study the relationship between CRF and fear. Takahashi (2001) reviewed the literature and identified three major methodological approaches including knock-out procedures, antisense oligonucleotide strategies and administration of a specific antagonists. The available data generally supports the implication of CRF1 in emotional behaviour. CRF2 also appears to be involved in the expression of both stress-induced and spontaneous anxiety behaviour, even though several inconsistencies are observable in the available studies. As pointed out by Takahashi (2001) the implication of both CRF1 and CRF2 in fear remains to be clarified and research evaluating the behavioural consequences of separate activation of the CRF receptor subtypes should be of particular relevance.

From Peptides to Emotional Interference: Opioïds and Cannabinoids

Even if the idea of a biochemical basis for emotion might by considered as untenable, there is clear evidence in the literature that peptides themselves are able to interfere with emotions. Opioïd peptides are an extensively studied example. Three classical families of opioïd peptides have been identified: enkephalines, endorphins and dynorphin. Each family is derived from a precursor polypeptide and has a characteristic anatomical distribution. The endogenous opioïd system is complex and subtle, holding great diversity (Gutstein and Akil, 2001) and only four identified opioïd receptors have been identified: Mu (Chen et al., 1993), Delta (Evans et al., 1992; Kieffer et al., 1992), Kappa (Yasuda et al., 1993; Meng et al., 1993) and Orphan (Libert et al., 1991; Bunzow et al., 1994; Mollereau et al., 1994). Several sub-classes have also identified: Epsilon (Schultz et al., 1979), Iota (Oka, 1980), Lambda (Grevel and Sadee, 1983) and Zeta (Zagon et al., 1989). Opioïd receptors are part of the G protein-coupled receptor family, like CRF. The opioïds produce various mood modifications, such as euphoria, a feeling of well-being, etc., and it has been accepted that these opioïd properties contribute to their chronic and compulsive use. Although the exact mechanisms through which the opioïds produce these mood alterations are not entirely elucidated, much data implicates the dopaminergic system within a cerebral circuit of rewards. The cerebral mechanisms implied in the processes of reinforcement of the opioïds can be distinguished from those implied in the physical dependence (Koob and Bloom, 1988). Much evidence indicates that, with regard to positive reinforcements, the dopaminergic system plays an important role particularl2Yin the meso-cortico-limbic system DA (Di Chiara 1992; Kreek et al., 2002). This system is composed of various structures which include the tegmento-ventral area, the nucleus accumbens, the prefrontal cortex, the amygdala and the septum. Drugs, and in particular opioïds, interfere with this system of reward and underline, at least in part, the loss of control and the compulsive need to consume. Various studies (Stolerman, 1992; Nicoll, 1980) indicate the opioïds' ability to interfere with dopaminergic transmission via the GABAergic system. Opioïds could inhibit the GABAergic neurons that allow the inhibition of the dopaminergic neurons in the tegmento ventral area. This effect of the opioïds on GABA is likely to involve a massive release of dopamine in the nucleus accumbens as well as in other parts of the limbic system (Johnson and North, 1992). However, dopamine is not the only element associated with the opioïds' reinforcing capacity, as indicated by studies where the suppression of the dopaminergic terminals in the nucleus accumbens does not induce an interruption of heroin auto-administration behaviour (Pettit et al., 1984). Data also indicates that the Mu receptor appears to be a determining factor in the reinforcing mechanisms of morphine (Matthes et al., 1996; Sora et al. 1997). Therefore, the Mu receptor plays a central part in the reinforcing effects of the opioïds whereas dopamine plays only a modest or, at best, secondary role (Kreek et al., 2002). The Mu receptor is involved in the reinforcing effects of other drugs and other systems are implied in the modulation of the effects of the opioïds (Ledent et al., 1999). This relationship between opioïds and other systems susceptible to interference in the expression of mood can be illustrated by cannabinoids. Delta 9 THC (THC hereafter), one of the exogenous ligands of the cannabinoid system, is frequently used as a modulator of mood. THC, the main mind-altering substance in cannabis, was identified by Mechoulam in 1964. Two cannabinoid receptors have also been identified: the CB1, present in brain and peripheral organs, and the CB2, mainly present in the immune system (Felder and Glass, 1998). Within the brain, CB1 receptors are clustered in the cerebral cortex (particularly in the frontal cortex), the hippocampus, the basal ganglia, the cerebellum and the nucleus accumbens (Streel et al., 2002). Two endogenous ligands are identified: archidonylethanolamide, known as anandamide and 2-arachydonylglycerol (2-AG). Opioïds and cannabinoids share several mechanisms and pharmacological properties (Dewey, 1986), both leading, for example, to analgesia (Lichtman and Martin, 1991). The relationship between opioïd and cannabinoid systems has been clearly highlighted by Ledent et al. (1999) using CB1 knock-out mice. They demonstrated that CB1 receptors may mediate some of the psychoactive properties of opiates and may also be involved in the development of physical dependence on opiates. Evidence of interaction between both systems has been confirmed (Meng et al., 1998; Piomelli et al., 2000). Nevertheless, other studies indicate that CB1 receptors do not appear to be involved in all responses to opiates; for example, pain response modulation by opiates does not seem to be affected by CB1 suppression (Cossu et al., 2001). As frequent inconsistencies between observed and expected results have been noted in knock-out mice, Mas-Nieto and al (2001) studied the behavioural changes classically observed following chronic opiate exposure in mice treated with the combination of morphine and SR 141716A, a CB1 antagonist. Their results showed that only long-term CB1 antagonist administration mimicking the situation encountered in CB1 knock-out mice, reduced development of physical morphine dependence. The effects of opiates are also modulated by other variables including substance P, another peptide. Murtra et al. (2000) showed, for example, that the physical response to opioïds was reduced in substance P knock-out mice. As the P substance receptor is found in large quantities in areas of the brain that are associated with depression, anxiety and stress, pharmacological modulation of substance P offers a radical new approach to these mood alterations (DeFelipe et al., 1998; Kramer et al., 1998; Culman et al., 1997). Together, these results highlight the role of specific systems, such as opioïds and cannabinoïds, in the modulation of mood while also indicating the potential capacity of endogenous and exogenous ligand (morphine, THC, ...) to interfere within these system leading to alterations in emotional states. Furthermore, recent results have indicated that the endogenous cannabinoid systems could control extinction of aversive memories (Marsicano et al., 2002). Aversive memories are acquired and stored in the central nervous system and, in the absence of reinforcement, the resulting behavioural response will gradually diminish till it is finally extinct (Marsicano et al., 2002). The integrity of the CB1 receptors seems to be required in the process of extinction. CB1 knock-out mice showed impaired short-term and long-term extinction in fear-conditioning, with unaffected memory acquisition and consolidation. The same results are observed using SR 141716A (CB1 antagonist). Therefore, Marsicano et al. (2002) proposed that stimulation of CB1 receptors could facilitate extinction of aversive memories through inhibitory networks in the amygdala. These results, if confirmed, could have an important impact in the management of different pathologies where fear plays a crucial role (e.g. post traumatic stress disorder). Furthermore, evidence of cannabis use by patients with psychiatric conditions can be construed as self-medication against the fear and anxiety associated with the early stages of psychiatric pathology, rather than as a contributory factor in the emergence of psychiatric illness.

From THC to Mood Alterations: A Psychiatric Perspective

Cannabis is one of the most widely used illicit drugs, with at least 45 million adults in the European Union having tried cannabis at some point in their lives (Rigter and van Laar, 2002). Cannabis consumption can be only understood by taking into account a range of personal, social and cultural characteristics. Most people do not take cannabis for long, using it mostly for recreational or experimental purposes (Rigter and van Laar, 2002). The psychoactive effects of THC are varied and depend on the users' expectations and/or mental state. Enhanced somatosensory perceptions are common and, at higher doses, auditory and visual hallucinations are described (Hanak et al., 2002; Weiss and Millman, 1998). Cantwell (2003) examined the association and effects of substance abuse in patients with a classical mood-altered pathology: schizophrenia. The results showed that patients with substance-use problems were younger, more likely to be male, and have a shorter duration of illness. Cannabis was the most commonly used drug, followed by opioïds. Dixon et al. (1990) interviewed 83 patients with schizophrenia. They found that patients who did not use cannabis were reported to be more suspicious and to suffer as many, if not more, hallucinations than patients using cannabis. Interestingly, more recent studies indicate abnormalities in the endocannabinoid system of patients with a diagnostic of schizophrenia (Leweke et al., 1999; Dean et al., 2001). The results of Dean and al (2001) indicated that there are changes in cannabinoid CB1 receptors in the dorsolateral prefrontal cortex that could prove to be associated with the pathology of schizophrenia. Schneider et al. (1998) provide evidence of strong similarities between data acquired from patients suffering from schizophrenia and THC intoxicated volunteers and, more recently, DeMarchi et al. (2003) showed that endocannabinoid signalling might be altered during the acute phase of schizophrenia. Nevertheless, the targeting of the cannabinoid systems in the treatment of psychosis (e.g. blockade of CB1 receptor) on its own appears insufficient for use in antipsychotic therapy. Therefore, even if the role of cannabinoid systems in psychiatric disorders such as schizophrenia seem to be obvious, further studies should investigate molecular and cellular mechanisms underlying this association. Overall, we need to better understand the opioïd and cannabinoid systems as new pharmacological interventions for the emotional disorders are likely to emerge from such research over the next few years.

From Psychological Disorder to Pharmacological Interventions Individual Susceptibilities

Fear and related concepts such as "anxiety" are normal adaptive phenomena and necessary to the survival of the species. However, adaptive functions can become inadequate, pathological, and/or interfere with the capacity to manage one's life. Various researchers have questioned the contribution of individual differences in the etiology such incapacity. As Steimer underlines (2002), Pavlov indicated that individual susceptibilities were not identical with regard to "experimental neuroses". The scientific literature indicates that in animals, anxiety is frequently associated with a genetic predisposition and with the influence of environmental factors. The genetic predisposition would be related to the types of genes present in the mechanisms underlying the expression of fear or anxiety. For example, in a case controlled study of the genetic polymorphism of three neurotransmitter system candidate genes, in patients with bipolar disorders with and without lifetime panic disorder, Rotondo et al. (2002) showed that bipolar disorder, with or without panic disorder, represents distinct genetic forms. Other data indicate that fear conditioning seems to result in selective gene expression in the basolateral amygdaloïd complex, supporting the idea that the amygdala is a site of neural plasticity and information storage during the formation of fear memory (Pape and Stork, 2003). Furthermore, Hettema et al. (2003) studied fear conditioning in 173 same-sex twin pairs (90 monozygotic and 83 dizygotic). Fear-relevant and fear-irrelevant sequences were used as conditioned stimuli paired with a mild electric shock (unconditioned stimulus). Their results showed that 2 sets of genes may underline the trait of fear conditioning while also providing evidence of differences in heritability based on the fear relevance of the stimulus. Together, these results indicate that genes represent a significant source of variation in the process of fear conditioning (Hettema et al., 2003). Environmental factors can interact with the expression of relevant genes during early development and determine the functional properties of the neural and biochemical systems involved in coping with stressful events (Steimer, 2002). Environmental factors can also modulate the learning process of coping strategies and determine the ability to cope successfully with any later threatening situations (Steimer, 2002). As an example, Fivush (2003) showed that parent-child reminiscing about negative experiences influenced the child's developing "emotional self-concept". Nevertheless, both common and fear-specific genes and common and fear-specific environments play important roles in the development of psychopathological expressions of emotions.

Neurobiological theories of personality also offer heuristic value in understanding emotional disorders. Such theories suggest that heritable or inborn defects in information processing, regulation of affect, and/or interpersonal behaviour are important in the aetiology of emotional disorders. For instance, Depue (1996) proposes that three major personality factors (specifiÙðlly, positive emotionality, negative emotionality and constraint), all associated with particular neurobiological systems, interact in the development of personality and, possibly, individual differences in susceptibility to emotional disorders. The dopamine system is thought to mediate positive emotionality which is related to incentive-reward motivation and active goal facilitation. Negative emotionality, conceptualised as a warning-alarm system aiming to facilitate the direction of attention under conditions of environmental uncertainty or threat, has been touted in animal studies to be associated with norepinephrine activity in the locus cereleus. Furthermore, animal studies of serotonin support its role in increasing the threshold for facilitation of behavioural and emotional response to stress. Each of these systems is seen to have a modulatory role in influencing the flow of information in neural networks. Cloninger (1987) similarly regards novelty seeking, harm avoidance and reward dependence to be related to dopamine, serotonin, and noradrenaline systems, respectively, and considers these central to development of emotional problems. While such approaches are viewed as important in improving our understanding of personality traits, it is unclear if the same neurobiological processes thought to underlie normal personality are functionally and structurally similar to those involved in pathology (Depue, 1996). Furthermore, the degree of dysfunction associated with particular personality patterns will depend to a great extent on contextual factors.

Cognitive theories of anxiety have also informed us about vulnerabilities to anxiety-based disorders. For example, obsessive-compulsive disorder has been associated with information processing and attentional biases (Kyrios and Iob, 1998), neuropsychological deficits

(Purcell, Maruff, Kyrios and Pantelis, 1998), and dysfunctional beliefs (Frost and Steketee, 2002; Riskin, Williams and Kyrios, 2002). While the biological substrates of these "deficits" remain elusive, their detailed description has been associated with the development of effective cognitive-behavioural treatments (Kyrios, 2003; Franklin and Foa, 1998). It is against such evidence-based psychological treatments for anxiety disorders that pharmacological treatments must be compared. In general, while genetic, cognitive, experiential and personality-based models all describe some important aspect or process of susceptibility to the pathological manifestation of fear, further studies certainly need to address their respective contributions. Nonetheless, purported neurobiological disruptions underlying disorder must be seen within environmental, developmental and experiential contexts which also influence the manifestation of behavior. While an arsenal of psychosocial strategies will always be necessary to deal effectively with the individual within his/her context, a neurobiological approach to individual susceptibility can provide future directions for the pharmacological treatment of emotional disorders.

Pharmacological Interventions

Emotional disturbances are extremely common in medical practice and in psychiatry (Baldessarini, 2001), from sadness to incapacitating illness where fear can be a major component (e.g. panic disorder). Symptoms of anxiety are seen across a range of disorders including panic disorder, generalised anxiety disorder, phobias, post-traumatic stress disorder, obsessive-compulsive disorder, and social anxiety disorder, as well as other conditions such as depression, dysthymia, adjustment disorders, and personality disorders (Baldessarini, 2001; Liebowitz, 1993). The present state of affairs in the treatment of anxiety and related disorders has been well summarised in various review papers and books (Barlow and Lehman, 1996; Nathan and Gorman, 1998), with both psychological and pharmacological treatments found to be effective. With regard to pharmacological treatments for panic, generalised anxiety disorder and phobic disorders, Roy-Burne and Cowley (1998) support the use of various tricyclic and serotinergic agents and benzodiazepines.

Historically, imipramine was the first effective pharmacological agent in the treatment of panic disorder (Ansseau and Sabbe, 2003). Clomipramine was also shown to be effective. Both imipramine and clomipramine require approximately a two-month treatment period before significant symptom amelioration is observed, although side effects have been considered a limiting factor in the widespread utility of these agents. More recently, due to their relatively safer side-effect profile and efficacy, serotonin reuptake inhibitors (SSRIs) have been considered as first choice in various pathologies where fear is omnipresent as it is the case in panic disorder. Monoamine oxydase agents are also frequently used on patients with associated depressive symptoms (Ansseau and Sabbe, 2003).

Currently, along with the SSRIs, benzodiazepines (BZD hereafter) are the most commonly employed treatment for clinical anxiety disorders (Baldessarini, 2001). Interestingly, although there has been concern about the potential for abuse with sedative medications like BZD, as well as concerns about the risk of cognitive impairment and falls with fractures associated with compromised motor skills (Ray et al., 1987), some studies suggest that physicians tend to be conservative and may even undertreat patient with anxiety (Baldessarini, 2001). The range of BZD induce qualitatively similar effects, but quantitative difference in their pharmacodynamic spectra is observable; hence, they have varying patterns of therapeutic applications. BZD produce their effect via the GABA receptor. With two subtypes of GABA receptors known as GABAa and GABAb, BZD do not activate directly GABAb receptors, but rather are considered allosteric modulators of GABAa receptors.. There are multiple molecular forms of BZD receptors, with at least five BZD receptors subtypes. Activation of BZD receptors underlie virtually all the desirable (e.g. anxiolytic effects) and undesirable (e.g. amnesic effect, development of dependence) pharmacological actions of BZD (Stahl, 2000). While some BZD (e.g. clonazepam) are effective in severe anxiety with strong autonomic overactivity (panic disorder) (Baldessarini, 2001), they appear to be less effective for generalized anxiety (Roerig 1999). Little evidence has been found for the effectiveness of particular BZDs with respect to specific subtypes of the same anxiety disorder. For instance, panic disorders subtype has been described (Briggs et al., 1993; Lelliot and Bass, 1990) according to the presence or absence of conspicuous respiratory symptoms. Valença et al. (2003) evaluated the difference in response to clonazepam in both subtypes of panic disorder. Their results showed that clonazepam had similar effect in the treatment of panic disorder patients with the respiratory and non-respiratory subtypes. Another class of agent with beneficial effects in anxiety treatment are the azapirones, represented clinically by buspirone (Buspar; Niman et al., 1998). Buspirone has selective affinity for serotonin receptors of the 5-HT1a type, for which it appears to be a partial agonist (Sanders-Bush and Mayer, 2001). Buspirone is not sedating, has few cognitive side effects and does¡,ot induce dependence (McCance-Katz and Kosten, 1998). However, while buspirone seems to be beneficial for some but not all anxious patients (McCance-Katz and Kosten, 1998; Ninan et al., 1998; Taylor, 1998), it lacks efficacy in severe anxiety with panic attacks (Baldessarini, 2001). Finally, as buspirone can take up to 4 weeks before it has any therapeutic effect, its usefulness in clinical practice is limited (McCance-Katz and Kosten, 1998).

As anxiety disorders are commonly associated with depression and dysthymia, use of treatments that are also effective in the treatment of affective disturbances is generally advantageous in clinical practice. Hence, tricyclics, SSRIs and evidence-based psychological treatments such as cognitive-behaviour therapy have some advantage over BZDs. Relapse rates following discontinuation of treatment are a further consiferation in the development of future treatments. While psychological treatments appear to work directly on vulnerability factors such as cognitions (Kyrios, Hordern and Bhar, 2003), pharmacological treatments need to establish therapeutic effects on factors that render individuals susceptible to anxiety disorders. Furthermore, as previously stated, anxiety-based conditions are frequently associated with substance abuse. Anxiety, fear, emotions and abuse of drugs present in a complex fashion to the clinician who must find a way through diagnostic dilemmas and decisions about treatment priorities. A large number of patients present with "dual diagnoses" and need to be treated keeping in mind the potential interaction between their use of drugs and prescribed medications. A further issue regarding the treatment of anxiety disorders concerns the combination of various treatments, whether such combinations constitute polypharmacy or a combined psychological/pharmacological treatment approach. Some medications (e.g. BZDs) may interfere with psychological retraining processes, while medication treatments in general may interfere with the development of adaptive attributions in anxious patients. On the other hand, psychological treatments may improve adherence to pharmacological treatments, thus enhancing outcomes. Of greatest concern for any treatment, however, is the potential emergence of aversive side effects which not only affect patients' quality of life, but ultimately influence drop-out rates.

CONCLUSIONS

Far away from earlier physiological and psychological considerations about emotions, basic neuroscience and animal research is now entering an era where researchers are trying to fill the gap between neurobiological discoveries and clinical practice. Emotions and fear are still, at least at the neurochemical level, poorly understood. While there is a huge accumulation of data, an integrative theory is still missing. Furthermore, available pharmacological strategies are still insufficient. However, peptides would appear to carry some hope in both understanding the underlying mechanisms of emotions and developing new pharmacological strategies. In order to modulate the response elicited by a peptide there are two distinct approaches. On the one hand, it is possible to use an exogenous agonist/antagonist that acts on peptide receptors (e.g. opioïd receptors). However, this technique is not without side effects and, as is the case with opioïds, chronic stimulation of the receptors leads to tolerance and dependence. On the other hand, it is also possible to modulate the extracellular levels of endogenous peptide effectors by inhibiting their metabolizing enzymes (Roques et al., 1993). Even if peptidase inhibitors have lower pharmacological potency in comparison to exogenous agonists (Roques, 2000) they could be of great interest in the management of fear-related symptoms. Accordingly, enkephalins protecting from metabolisation have been shown to be active in all tests used to screen anti-depressant drugs (Roques, 2000). Opioïd and cannabinoid systems are in a functional relationship, therefore available modulators of extracellular concentration of endogenous opioïds could interfere with fear-like symptoms, especially when one considers the role of the cannabinoid system in aversive memory (Marsicanno et al., 2002). However, in the development of new medications such as peptide inhibitors, researchers will have to face new problems such as genetic variability in drug-response. As pointed out by Roques (2000), more than two decades were required to identify the tachykinin NK1 receptor agonist as a new approach to depression (Kramer et al., 1998). Regarding the growing number of teams involved in the study of emotions, it should take less time for researchers to specify the potential association between peptide modulation and the expression of emotions, thus leading to a new era of more efficient therapeutic approaches in the management of emotions and/or fear related symptoms. However, such research needs to integrate current knowledge and theories about individual vulnerability to the development of anxiety disorders. Future pharmacological developments will need to be assimilated into the complex realities of clinical practice where the patient's experiential context is the basic unit on which clinicians exert creative influence. Issues such as adherence, drop out, and relapse rates will need to be dealt with, as will the degree to which pharmacological agents are effective in changing individual vulnerabilities following discontinuation of active treatment. These sorts of challenges are not specific to the area of anxiety, but form a necessary part of all ongoing clinically-based research.

REFERENCES

Ansseau, M., and Sabbe, B. (2003).Troubles anxieux. In M. Dierick, M. Ansseau, H. D'haenen, J. Peuskens, and P. Linkowski (Eds). *Manuel de Psychopharamcothérapie* (pp. 231-276). Gent: Academia Press.

Baldessarini, R. (2001). Drugs and the treatment of psychiatric disorders: depression and anxiety disorders. In J. Hardman, L. Limbird, and A. Goodman-Giman (Eds). *The Pharmacological basis of Therapeutics -10th ed.* (pp. 447-483). New-York: McGraw-Hill.

Barlow, D.H. and Lehman, C.L. (1996). Advances in the psychosocial of anxiety disorders: Implications for national healthcare. *Archives of General Psychiatry, 53,* 727-735.

Bear, M., Connors, B., and Paradiso, M. (1997). *Neurosciences à la découverte du cerveau.* Paris: Masson.

Blair, H.T., Schafe, G.E., Bauer, E.P., Rodrigues, S.M., and LeDoux, J.E. (2001). Synaptic plasticity in the lateral amygdala: a cellular hypothesis of fear conditioning. *Learn. Mem., 8(5),* 229-42.

Blanchard, C., Blanchard, R., Fellous, J.M., Guismaraes, F.S., Irwin, W., LeDoux, J.E., McGaugh, J.L., Rosen, J.B., Schenberg, L.C., Volchan, E., and Da Cunha, C. (2001). The brain decade in debate: III. Neurobiology of emotion. *Braz. J. Med. Biol. Res., 34(3),* 283-293.

Bloom, F. (2001). Neurotransmission and the central nervous system. In J. Hardman, L. Limbird, and A. Goodman-Gilman (Eds). *The Pharmacological basis of Therapeutics - 10th ed.* (pp.293-320). New-York: McGraw-Hill.

Briggs, A.C., Streetch, D.D., and Brandon, S. (1993). Subtyping of panic disorder by symptom profile. *Br. J. Psychiatry, 163,* 201-209.

Bunzow, J.R., Saez, C., Mortrud M., Bouvier, C., Williams, J.T., Low, M., and Grandy, D.K. (1994). Molecular cloning and tissue distribution of a putative member of the rat opioid receptor gene family that is not a μ, _, _ opioid receptor type. *FEBS Lett., 347,* 284-288.

Cahill, L., Weinberger, N.M., Roozendaal, B., and McGaugh, J.L. (1999). Is the amygdala a locus of "conditioned fear"? Some questions and caveats. *Neuron, 23,* 227-228.

Cantwell, R. (2003). Scottish1 omorbidity Study Group. Substance use and schizophrenia: effects on symptoms, social functioning and service use. *Br. J. Psychiatry, 182,* 324-9.

Cardoso, S.H., Melo, L.L., Coimbra, N.C., and Brandao, M.L. (1992). Opposite effects of low and high doses of morphine on neuronal substrates of aversion in the inferior colliculus. *Behav. Pharmacol., 3,* 489-495.

Chang, C.P., Pearse II, R.V., O'Connell, S., and Rosenfeld, M.G. (1993). Identification of a seven transmembrane helix receptor for corticotropin-releasing factor and sauvagine in mammalian brain. *Neuron, 11,* 1187-1195.

Chen, Y., Mestek, A., Liu, J., Hurley, J.A., and Yu, L. (1993). Molecular cloning and fonctional expression of a mu-opioid receptor from rat brain. *Mol. Pharmaco., 44,* 8-12.

Cloninger, C.R. (1987). A systematic method for clinical description and classification of personality variants: A proposal. *Archives of General Psychiatry, 44,* 573 – 588.

Coimbra, N.C., and Brandao, M.L. (1993). GABAergic nigro-collicular pathways modulate the defensive behaviour elicited by midbrain tectum stimulation. *Behav. Brain Res., 59,* 131-139.

Coimbra, N.C., and Brandao, M.L. (1997). Effects of 5-HT_2 receptors blockade on fear-induced analgesia elicited by electrical stimulation of the deep layers of the superior colliculus and dorsal periaqueductal gray matter. *Behav. Brain Res., 87,* 97-103.

Cossu, G., Ledent, C., Fattore, L., Imperato, A., Böhme, G.A., Parmentier, M., and Fratta, W. (2001). Cannabinoid CB_1 receptor knockout mice fail to self-administer morphine but not other drugs of abuse. *Behav. Brain Res., 118(1),* 61-65.

Coupland, N. (2000). Brain mechanisms and neurotransmitters. In D. Nutt, J. Davidson and J. Zohar (Eds). *Post-Traumatic Stress Disorder: Diagnosis, Managment and Treatment.* London: Martin Dunitz Ltd.

Cousens, G., and Otto, T. (1998). Both pre- and post-training excitotoxic lesions of the basolateral amygdala abolish the expression of olfactory and contextual fear conditioning. *Behav. Neurosci., 112,* 1092-1103.

Culman, J., Klee, S., Ohlendorf, C., and Unger, T. (1997). Effect of tachykinin receptor inhibition in the brain on cardiovascular and behavioural responses to stress. *J. Pharmacol. Exp. Ther., 280,* 238-246.

Damasio, A.R. (1994). *Descartes' Error. Emotion, Reason, and the human brain.* New-York: Putnam Book.

Darwin, C. (1872). *The Expression of Emotions in Man and Animals.* London: John Murray.

Davis, M. (1994). The role of the amygdala in emotional learning. *Int. Rev. Neurobiol., 36,* 225-266.

Dean, B., Sundram, S., Bradbury, R., Scarr, E., and Copolov, D. (2001). Studies on [3H]CP-55940 binding in the human central nervous system: regional specific changes in density of cannabinoid-1 receptors associated with schizophrenia and cannabis use. *Neuroscience, 103(1),* 9-15.

DeFelipe, C., Herrero, J.F., O'brien, J.A., Palmer, J.A., Doyle, C.A., Smith, A.J.H., Laird, J.M.A., Belmonte, C., Cervero, F., and Hunt, S.P. (1998). Altered nociception, analgesia and aggression in mice lacking the receptor for substance P. *Nature, 392,* 394-397.

Dejerine, J., and Gauckler, R. (1911). *Les Manifestations Fonctionnelles des Psychonévroses – leur traitement par la psychothérapie.* Paris: Masson.

DeMarchi, N., De Petrocellis, L., Orlando, P., Daniele, F., Fezza, F., and Di Marzo, V. (2003). Endocannabinoid signalling in the blood of patients with schizophrenia. *Lipids Health Dis., 2(1),* 5.

Depue, R.A. (1996). A neurobiological framework for the structure of personality and emotion: Implications for Personality Disorders. In Clarkin, J.F. and Lenzenweger, M.F. (Eds.) *Major Theories of Personality Disorder* (pp. 347- 390). New York: Guilford Press.

Dewey, W.L. (1986). Cannabinoid pharmacology. *Pharmacol. Rev., 38,* 151-178.

Di Chiara, G., and North, R.A. (1992). Neurobiology of opiate abuse. *Trends Pharmacol. Sci., 13(5),* 185-193.

Dixon, L., Haas, G., Weiden, P., Sweeney, J., and Frances, A. (1990). Acute effects of drug abuse in schizophrenic patients: clinical observations and patients' self-reports. *Schizophr. Bull., 16(1),* 69-79.

Eichenberger, G.C., Ribeiro, S.J., Osaki, M.Y., Maruoka, R.Y., Resende, G.C., Castellan-Baldan, L., Correa, S.A., Da Silva, L.A., and Coimbra, N.C. (2002). Neuroanatomical and psychopharmacological evidence for interaction between opioid and GABAergic neural pathways in the modulation of fear and defense elicited by electrical and chemical stimulation of the deep layers of the superior colliculus and dorsal periaqueductal gray matter. *Neuropharmacology, 42(1)*, 48-59.

Ekman, P. (1992). An argument for basic emotions. *Cognition and Emotions, 6,* 169-200.

Evans, C.J., Keith, D.E., Morrison, H., Magendzo. K., and Edwards, R.H. (1992). Cloning of a delta receptor by functional expression. *Science, 258,* 1952-55.

Eysenck, M. (1992). *Anxiety: The Cognitive Perspective.* Hove (UK): Lawrence Erlbaum Associates, Publishers.

Fanselow, M.S., and LeDoux, J.E. (1999). Why we think plasticity underlying Pavlovian fear conditioning occurs in the basolateral amygdala? *Neuron, 23,* 229-232.

Felder, C.C., and Glass, M. (1998). *Annu. Rev. Pharmacol. Toxicol., 38,* 179-200.

Fivush, R., Berlin, L.J., Sales, J.M., Mennuti-Washburn, J., and Cassidy, J. (2003). Functions of parent-child reminiscing about emotionally negative events. *Memory, 11(2)*, 179-92.

Franklin, M.E. and Foa, E. (1998). Cognitive-behavioural treatments for Obsessive-Compulsive Disorder. In P.E. Nathan and J.M. Gordon (Eds.) *A Guide to Treatments That Work* (pp. 339 – 357). Oxford: Oxford University Press.

Frijda, N. (1989). *The Emotions*. Cambridge: CUP.

Frost and G. Steketee (Eds.), *Cognitive approaches to obsessions and compulsions: Theory, assessment, and treatment.* Oxford: Elsevier

Graeff, F.G. (1990). Brain defense systems and anxiety. In M. Roth, G.D. Burrow, and R. Noyes (Eds.), *Handbook of Anxiety,* vol 3 (pp. 307-354). New-York: Elsevier.

Grevel, J., and Sadee, W. (1983). An opiate binding site in the rat brain is highly selective for 4.5-epoxymorphinans. *Science, 221,* 1198-1201.

Gutstein, H.B., and Akil, H. (2001). Opioid analgesics. In J. Hardman, L. Limbird, and A. Goodman-Giman (Eds). *The Pharmacological basis of Therapeutics -10th ed.* (pp. 569-619). New-York: McGraw-Hill.

Hanak, C., Tecco, J., Verbanck, P., and Pelc, I. (2002). Cannabis, mental health and dependence. In *Cannabis 2002 Report* (pp. 63-77). Ministry of health Belgium.

Hettema, J.M., Annas, P., Neale, M.C., Kendler, K.S., and Fredrikson, M. (2003). A twin study of the genetics of fear conditioning. *Arch. Gen. Psychiatry, 60(7)*, 702-8.

Hongjoo, L., and Jeansok, J.K. (1998). Amygdalar NMDA receptors are critical for new fear learning in previously fear-conditioned rats. *J. Neurosci., 18(20),* 8444-54.

Isaacson, R.L. (1982). *The Limbic System.* New-York: Plenum.

Johnson, S.W., and North, N.A. (1992). Opioids excite dopamine neurons by hyperpolarization of local interneurons. *J. Neurosci., 12(2),* 483-488.

Kieffer, B.L., Beford, K., Gaveriaux-Ruff, C., and Hirth, C.G. (1992). The delta-opioid receptor: isolation of a cDNA by expression cloning and pharmacological characterization. *Proc. Natl. Acad. Sci. U S A, 89,* 12048-12052.

Kim, M., and Davies, M. (1993). Electrolytic lesions of the amygdala block acquisition and expression of fear-potentiated startle even with extensive training but do not prevent reacquisition. *Behav. Neurosci., 107,* 580-595.

Koob, G.F., and Bloom, F.E. (1988). Cellular and molecular mechanisms of drug dependence. *Science, 242,* 715-723.

Kotter, R., and Meyer, N. (1992). The limbic system: a review of its empirical foundation. *Behav. Brain Res., 52(2),* 105-127.

Kramer, M.S., and al. (1998). Distinct mechanism for antidepressant activity by blockade of central substance P receptors. *Science, 281,* 1640-1645.

Kreek, M.J., La Forge, K.S., and Butelman, E. (2002). Pharmacotherapy of addictions. *Natl. Rev. Drug Discov., 1(9),* 710-726.

Kyrios, M. (2003). Exposure and response prevention in the treatment of Obsessive–Compulsive Disorder. In R. Menzies and P. de Silva (Eds.). *Obsessive-Compulsive Disorder: Theory, Research and Treatment* (pp. 259 – 274). Chichester, England: John Wiley and Sons.

Kyrios, M., Hordern, C. and Bhar, S. (2003). Cognitive changes in Obsessive-Compulsive Disorder following cognitive-behavior therapy. Paper presented at the Annual Conference of the Australian Association of Cognitive-Behaviour Therapy, Adelaide, Australia.

Kyrios, M. and Iob, M. (1998). Automatic and strategic processing in Obsessive-Compulsive Disorder: Attentional bias, cognitive avoidance or more complex phenomena?, *Journal of Anxiety Disorders, 12,* 271 – 292.

Ledent, C., Valverde, O., Cossu, G., Pettitet, F., Aubert, J.F., Beslot, F., Bohme, G.A., Imperato, A., Pedrazzini, T., Roques, B.P., Vassart, G., Fratta, W., and Parmentier, M. (1999). Unresponsiveness to cannabinoids and reduced addictive effects of opiates in CB1 receptor knockout mice. *Science, 283,* 5400-4.

LeDoux, J.E. (1991). Emotion and the limbic system concept. *Concepts Neurosci., 2,* 169-199.

LeDoux, J.E. (1993). Emotional memory: in search of systems and synapses. *Ann. NY Acad. Sci., 702,* 149-157.

LeDoux, J.E. (1994). Emotion, memory and the brain. *Sci. Am., 270,* 50-57.

LeDoux, J.E. (2000). Emotion circuits in the brain. *Annu. Rev. Neurosci., 23,* 155-84.

Lee, Y., Walker, D., and Davis, M. (1996). Lack of temporal gradient of retrograde amnesia following NMDA-induced lesions of the basolateral amygdala assessed with the fear-potentiated startle paradigm. *Behav. Neurosci., 110,* 836-839.

Lelliot, P., and Bass, C. (1990). Symptom specificity in patients with panic. *Br. J. Psychiatry, 157,* 593-597.

Leweke, F.M., Giuffrida, A., Wurster, U., Emrich, H.M., and Piomelli, D. (1999). Elevated endogenous cannabinoids in schizophrenia. *Neuroreport, 10(8),* 1665-9.

Libert, F., Schiffmann, S.N., Lefort, A., Parmentier, M., Gerard, C., Dumont, J.E., Vanderhaeghen, J.J., and Vassart, G. (1991). The orphan receptor cDNA RDC7 encodes an A1 adenosine receptor. *EMBO J., 10(7),* 1677-82.

Lichtman, A.H., and Martin, B.R. (1991). Spinal and supraspinal components of cannabinoid-induced antinociception. *J. Pharmacol. Exp. Ther., 258,* 517-523.

Liebowitz, M.R. (1993). Pharmacological treatment of social phobia: Traditional MAOIs and moclobemide. *European Neuropsychopharmacology, 3(3),* 193-194.

Lovenberg, T.W., Chalmers, D.T., Liu, C., and De Souza, E.B. (1995). $CRF_{2\_}$ and $CRF_{2\_}$ receptor mRNAs are differentially distributed between the rat central nervous system and peripheral tissues. *Endocrinology, 136,* 4139-4142.

Lynch, G. (1986). *Synapses, Circuits, and the Beginnings of Memory.* Cambridge, MA: MIT Press.

MacLean PD (1949). Psychosomatic disease and the " visceral brain ": recent developments bearing on the papez theory of emotion. *Psychosom. Med. 11,* 338-353.

MacLean, P.D. (1952). Some psychiatric implications of physiological studies on fronto-temporal portion of limbic system (visceral brain). *Clin. Neurphysiol., 4,* 407-418.

Maren, S. Aharonov, G., Stote, D.L., and Fanslow, M.S. (1996). N-methyl-d-aspartate receptors in the basolateral amygdala are required for both acquisition and expression of the conditional fear in rats. *Behav. Neurosci., 110,* 1365-1374.

Maren, S. (1998). Overtraining does not mitigate contextual fear conditioning deficits produced by neurotoxic lesions of the basolateral amygdala. *J. Neurosci., 18(8),* 3088-97.

Maren, S. (1999). Neurotoxic basolateral amygdala lesions impair learning and memory but not the performance of conditional fear in rats. *J. Neurosci., 19(19),* 8696-703.

Marsicano, G., Wotjak, C.T., Azad, S.C., Bisogno, T., Rammes, G., Cascio, M.G., Hermann, H., Tang, J., Hofmann, C., Zieglgansberger, W., Di Marzo, V., and Lutz, B. (2002). The endogenous cannabinoid system controls extinction of aversive memories. *Nature, 418(6897),* 530-4.

Mas-Nieto, M., Pommier, B., Tzavara, E.T., Caneparo, A., Da Nascimento, S., Le Fur, G., Roques, B.P., and Noble, F. (2001). Reduction of opioid dependence by the CB_1 antagonist SR141716A in mice: evaluation of the interest in pharmacotherapy of opioid addiction. *Br. J. Pharmacol., 132(8),* 1809-16.

Matthes, H.W., Maldonado, R., Simonin, F., Valverde, O., Slowe, S., Kitchen, I., Befort, K., Dierich, A., Le Meur, M., Dolle, P., Tzavara, E., Hanoune, J., Roques, B.P., and Kieffer, B.L. (1996). Loss of morphine-induced analgesia, reward effect and withdrawal symptoms in mice lacking the mu-opioid-receptor gene. *Nature, 383(6603),* 819-823.

McCance-Katz, E.F., and Kosten, T.R. (1998). *New Treatments for Chemical Addictions.* Washington: American Psychiatric Press.

McGaugh, J.L. (2000). Memory – a century of consolidation. *Science, 287,* 248-251.

Meng, F., Xie, G.X., Thompson, R.C., Mansour, A., Watson, S.J., and Akil, H. (1993). Cloning and pharmacological characterization of a rat kappa opioid receptor. *Proc. Natl. Acad. Sci. U S A, 90,* 9954-9958.

Meng, I.D., Manning, B.H., Martin, W.J., and Fields, H.L. (1998). An analgesia circuit activated by cannabinoids. *Nature, 395,* 381-383.

Miserendino, M.J., Sananes, C.B., Melia, K.R., and Davis, M. (1990). Blocking of acquisition but not expression of conditioned fear-potentiated startle by NMDA antagonists in the amygdala. *Nature, 345(6277),* 716-8.

Mollereau, C., Parmentier, M., Mailleux, P., Butour, J.L., Moisand, C., Chalon, P., Caput, D., Vassart, G., and Menier, J.C. (1994). ORL1, a novel member of the opioid receptor family. Cloning, functional expression and localization. *FEBS Lett., 341,* 33-38.

Mueser, K., Noordsy, D., Drake, R., and Fox, L. (2003). *Integrated Treatment for Dual Disorders.* New York – London: Guilford Press.

Murtra, P., Sheasby, A.M., Hunt, S.P., and De Felipe, C. (2000). Rewarding effects of opiates are absent in mice lacking the receptor for substance P. *Nature, 405(6783),* 180-3.

Nathan, P.E. and Gorman, J.M. (1997). *A Guide to Treatments That Work,* Oxford Uni Press.

Nicoll, R.A., Alger, B.E., and Jahr, C.E. (1980). Enkephalin blocks inhibitory pathways in the vertebrate CNS. *Nature, 287(5777),* 22-25.

Ninan, P.T., Cole, J.O., and Yonkers, K.A. (1998). Nonbenzodiazepine anxiolytics. In A.F. Schatzberg, and C.B Nemeroff (Eds). *The American Psychiatric Press Textbook of Psychopharmacology, 2nd ed.* (pp.287-300). Washington: American Psychiatric Press.

Oka, T. (1980). Enkephalin receptor in the rabbit ileum. *Life Sci., 38,* 1889-1898.

Pape, H.C., and Stork, O. (2003). Genes and mechanisms in the amygdala involved in the formation of fear memory. *Ann. N.Y. Acad. Sci., 985,* 92-105.

Pavlov, J. (1904). Sur la réaction psychique des glandes salivaires (phénomènes nerveux complexes dans le travail des glandes salivaires) [6123138] [Q372], *Archives Internationale de Physiologie, 1,* 119-135.

Pert, B. (1997). *Molecules of Emotion*. New York: Touchstone.

Pettit, H.O., Ettenberg, A., Bloom, F.E., and Koob, G.F. (1984). Destruction of dopamine in the nucleus accumbens selectively attenuates cocaine but not heroin self-administration in rats. *Psychopharmacol., 84,* 167-173.

Piomelli, D., Giuffrida, A., Calignano, A., and Rodriguez de Fonseca, F. (2000). The endocannabinoid system as a target for therapeutic drugs. *Trends Pharamacol; Sci., 21,* 218-224.

Purcell, R., Maruff, P., Kyrios, M. and Pantelis, C. (1998). Neuropsychological deficits in Obsessive-Compulsive Disorder: A comparison with Unipolar Depression, Panic Disorder, and Normal Controls. *Archives of General Psychiatry, 55*, 415 – 423.

Quirk, G.J., Repa, J.C., and LeDoux, J.E. (1995). Fear conditioning enhances short-latency auditory responses of lateral amygdala neurons: parallel recordings in the freely behaving rat. *Neuron, 15,* 1029-1039.

Quirk, G.J., Armony, J.L., and LeDoux, J.E. (1997). Fear conditioning enhances different temporal components of toned-evoked spike trains in auditory cortex and lateral amygdale. *Neuron, 19,* 613-624.

Radulovic, J., Rühmann, A., Liepold, T., and Spiess, J. (1999). Modulation of learning and anxiety by cortico-releasing factor (CRF) and stress: differential roles of CRF receptors 1 and 2. *J. Neurosc., 19,* 5016-5025.

Rigter, H., and van Laar, M. (2002). Epidemiological aspects of cannabis use. In *Cannabis 2002 Report* (pp.19-45). Ministry of health Belgium.

Riskind, J.H., Williams, N.L. and Kyrios, M. (2002). Experimental methods for studying cognition in Obsessive-Compulsive Disorder. In: R. O. Frost and G. Steketee (Eds.), *Cognitive approaches to obsessions and compulsions: Theory, assessment, and treatment* (pp. 139 – 164). Oxford: Elsevier.

Roerig, J. L. (1999). Diagnosis and management of generalized anxiety disorder. *J. Am. Pharm. Assoc. (Wash)., 39(6),* 811-21.

Roques, B.P., and al., (1993). Neutral endopeptidase 24.11: structure, inhibition, and experimental and clinical pharmacology. *Pharmacol. Rev., 45,* 87-146.

Roques, P.R. (2000). Novel approaches to targeting neuropeptide systems. *TiPS, 21,* 475-483.

Rotondo, A., Mazzanti, C., Dell'Osso, L., Rucci, P., Sullivan, P., Bouanani, S., Gonnelli, C., Goldman, D., and Cassano, G. B. (2002). Catechol o-methyltransferase, serotonin transporter, and tryptophan hydroxylase gene polymorphisms in bipolar disorder patients with and without comorbid panic disorder. *Am. J. Psychiatry, 159(1),* 23-9.

Roy-Burne, P.P and Cowley, D.S. (1998). Pharmacological treatment of panic, generalised anxiety and phobic disorders. In Nathan, P.E. and Gorman, J.M. (Eds.) *A Guide to Treatments That Work* (pp. 319 – 338). Oxford Uni Press.

Sanders-Bush, E., and Mayer, S.E. (2001). 5-Hydroxytryptamine (serotonin): receptor agonists and antagonists. In J.G. Hardman, L.E. Limbird, and A. Goodman Gilman (Eds). *The Pharmacological basis of Therapeutics. -10th ed.* (pp. 269-290). New-York: McGraw-Hill.

Schmitt, P., Carrive, P., DiScala, G., Jenck, F., Brandao, M.L., Bagri, A., Moreau, J.L., and Sandner, G. (1986). A neuropharmacological study of the periventricular neural substrate involved in flight. *Behav. Brain Res., 22,* 181-190.

Schneider, U., Leweke, F.M., Mueller,-Vahl, K.R., and Emrich, H.M. (1998). Cannabinoid/anandamide system and schizophrenia: is there evidence for association? *Pharamacopsychiatry, 31(2),* 110-113.

Schulz, R., Faase, E., Wuster, M., and Herz, A. (1979). Selective receptors for beta-endorphin on the rat vas deferens. *Life Sci., 24,* 843-849.

Scoville, W.B., and Milner, B. (1957). Loss of recent memory after bilateral hippocampal lesions. *J. Neurol. Psychol., 20,* 11-21

Sora, I., Takahashi, N., Funada, M., Ujike, H., Revay, R.S., Donovan, D.M., Miner, L.L., and Uhl, G.R. (1997). Opiate receptor knockout mice define mu receptor roles in endogenous nociceptive responses and morphine-induced analgesia. *Proc. Natl. Acad. Sci. U S A, 94,* 1544-49.

Stahl, S.M. (2000). *Essential Psychopharmacology. Neuroscientific basis and Practical Applications*. Cambridge: University Press.

Steimer, T. (2002). The biology of fear and anxiety-related behaviours. *Dial. Clin. Neurosci., 4 (3),* 231-249.

Stolerman, I. (1992). Drugs of abuse: behavioral principles, methods and terms. *Trends Pharmacol. Sci., 13(5),* 170-176.

Streel, E., Verbanck, P., and Pelc, I. (2002). Pharmacology and neurobiological aspects of cannabis. In *Cannabis 2002 Report* (pp.47-53). Ministry of health Belgium.

Takahashi, L.K. (2001). Role of CRF(1) and CRF(2) receptors in fear and anxiety.*Neurosci. Biobehav. Rev., 25(7-8)*, 627-36.

Tang, J., Wagner, S., Schachner, M., Dityatev, A., and Wotjak, C.T. (2003). Potentiation of amygdaloid and hippocampal auditory-evoked potentials in a discriminatory fear-conditioning task in mice as a function of tone pattern and context. *European Journal of Neuroscience, 18,* 639-650.

Tao, R., and Auerbach, S.B. (2000). Regulation of serotonin release by GABA and excitatory amino acids. *J. Psychopharm., 14,* 100-113.

Vaillant, G.E. (2003). Mental health. *Am. J. Psychiatry, 160(8)*, 1373-84.

Valenca, A.M., Nardi, A.E., Mezzasalma, M.A., Nascimento, I., Zin, W.A., Lopes, F.L., and Versiani, M. (2003). Therapeutic response to benzodiazepine in panic disorder subtypes. *Sao Paulo Med. J., 121(2)*, 77-80.

Vazdarjanova, A., and McGaugh, J.L. (1998). Basolateral amygdale is not critical for congnitive memory of contextual fear conditioning. *Proc. Natl. Acad. Sci. U S A, 95,* 15003-15007.

Weiss, C., and Millman, R. (1998). Hallucinogens, phencyclidine, marijuana, inhalants. In R. frances, and S. Miller (Eds.), *Cinical Textbook of Addictive Disorders*. New York: Guilford Press.

Yasuda, K., Raynor, K., Kong, H., Breder, C.D., Reisene, T., and Bell, G.I. (1993). Cloning and functional comparison of kappa and delta opioid receptor from mice brain. *Proc. Natl. Acad. Sci. U S A, 90,* 6736-6740.

Zagon, I.S., Goodman, S.R., and McLaughlin, J. (1989). Characterization of zeta: a new opioid receptor involved in growth. *Brain. Res., 482(2),* 297-305.

In: Fear in Cognitive Neuroscience
Editor: Salvatore Campanella, pp. 117-155
ISBN: 1-59454-502-2

Chapter 6

FEAR AND ANXIETY IN PSYCHIATRIC DISORDERS, COGNITIVE-BEHAVIORAL CONCEPTS AND TREATMENTS

***A. Velardi*[*1], *R. Willis*[2] *and V. Pomini*[3]**

[1] Unité Hospitalière Médico-psychologique. Hôpital régional de Delémont. Fbg. des Capucins 30, 2800 Delémont, Suisse.

[2] Institutions Psychiatriques du Valais Romand, Rue Saint Guérin 3, 1950 Sion, Suisse.

[3] Unité d'Enseignement des Thérapies Comportementales et cognitives. Institut de psychothérapie. Département Universitaire de Psychiatrie Adulte. Bâtiment des Cèdres, Site de Cery, 1008 Prilly-Lausanne, Suisse

1. INTRODUCTION

Who has never been afraid? No one without a doubt; fear being such an integral part of existence. Fear is essential to the survival of the species because it helps to identify and avoid dangers that can compromise existence. Everyone recognizes the necessity of fear; even if it is an unpleasant experience we prefer avoiding. And when fear no longer has an object, when it is prolonged without any apparent reason and progressively invades an individual's daily life until he can't work, go out or meet other people, it ends up loosing its functional aspect and usefulness: fear then becomes a disease.

Anxiety disorders have the highest prevalence among psychiatric illnesses. Global prevalence per year for all the anxiety disorders oscillates between 8% and 16% according to different studies; the prevalence in a lifetime can be as high as 20% (Bijl, Ravelli, and van Zessen, 1988; Goldberg and Lecrubier, 1995; Magee, Eaton, Wittchen, McGonagle, and Kessler, 1996). However the actual figure is certainly much higher, because there is practically no psychiatric disorder where anxiety doesn't play a role, even if it isn't the primary symptom. Anxiety currently appears as one of the most frequent psychological

[*] Email: alfredo.velardi@cgh.ch

problems psychiatrists encounter in their practice. Our modern society spends billions of dollars every year on anxiolytic medications (Barlow, 1988), and even more if one counts all forms of therapy, psychotherapy, methods of personal development and also the use of somatic health services (Rees, Richards, and Smith, 1988). Anxiety represents a habitual cause for medical visits, much higher than the rate for colds, coughs, influenza and other minor illnesses (Marsland, Wood, and Mayo, 1976). It also constitutes a frequent source of work absenteeism (Laitinen-Krispijn and Bijl, 2000). Hence, in its sub-pathological and pathological forms, fear represents an important issue for public health and for personal well-being.

As disciplines mainly interested in psychological and mental problems, psychiatry and psychotherapy have developed numerous categorizations and conceptualizations of anxiety disorders. Various types of treatment have also been derived from these theories. Entire volumes have been devoted to this topic, and it would of course be impossible here to synthesize all the various existing approaches used to understand and treat these illnesses. We have therefore chosen to concentrate on one particular psychotherapeutic approach, the cognitive-behavioral therapy (CBT). This treatment has gained so much theoretical and empirical support through the years that it is now recognized as one of the most effective methods to treat this syndrome (Grawe, Donate, and Bernauer, 1994; Kipta, Lueger, Saunders, and Howard, 1999). Let us describe this kind of recommended treatment and its theoretical background.

2. Fear and Anxiety

Fear is one of the basic emotions; other being disgust, joy, sadness, anger and surprise (Ekman, 1994; Ortony and Turner, 1990). Characterized by highly negative affect and physiologic excitation, this emotion appears in situations of danger. It informs of the presence of danger and prepares the organism to face it or to escape (Barlow, 1988).

Fear can vary in intensity: from slight apprehension to extremely intolerable panic. It can take miscellaneous forms where fearful thoughts and bodily reactions are each expressed with more or less intensity. Dangers which produce fear can be real (for example fear experienced during an accident, a catastrophe, an aggression, etc.), but also completely imaginary. In that case fear arouses from the meanings that the individual gives to a situation: fear appears because the person considers the situation as dangerous for him, even though it may not the case. Classically these specific and unfounded fears are called phobias. They most often concern animals (pets, insects), night or darkness, burglars, thunder etc. Simple or multiple phobias are frequent in childhood and have a tendency to disappear with age (Gray, 1991). Phobias of a crowd, open or closed areas (for example public places, restaurants, cinemas, tunnels, elevators, planes, etc.) are grouped under the term agoraphobia. In social phobias the individual is afraid of other people, in particular when the contact with others implies a particular performance (speaking in public, eating at an official dinner, exams, defending one's own rights, making requests, etc.) or the judgement of others. Fear can also be generalized to nearly the entire experience of life. In generalized anxiety disorders indeed preoccupations are no longer focalized on one or a few objects/situations, but can touch upon virtually all domains of existence (social life, social relationships, work, leisure, etc.): mere decisions or routine activities are seen by the person as insuperable obstacles and become instead numerous sources of anxiety. Post-traumatic stress disorders are another pathological form of expression of fear and anxiety. Normally one can experience anxiety and fear during a real traumatizing experience; these emotions can also occur after the trauma (after a few hours, days, weeks or months): compared to phobias, these fears originate from a terrible event that actually happened (violence, sexual abuse, accident, risk of imminent death, etc.). In the case of post-traumatic stress disorder they continue to persist in the absence of any danger. Here, the reasons for fear are no longer a current, future or imaginary danger. On the contrary, they concern the past and they unexpectedly haunt the person during the day as well as the night in the form of flashbacks, nightmares, irritability and anxiety among other symptoms that can last for years.

Even though the phobias evoked up to this point are irrational (because they don't warn of a current or real danger), they remain partially understandable. They can virtually become totally delusional. This is the case for example in psychoses or obsessive-compulsive disorders. Individuals affected by these illnesses sometimes present very strange fears: psychotic patients, for example, can develop the fear that they will be victims of a divine punishment or of a wicked plot against them; in obsessional compulsive disorder, different fears such as being contaminated by filth, being the cause of accidents harming others through negligence, or even committing blasphemies are very current.

2.1. The Distinction Between Fear and Anxiety

It is classic to theoretically distinguish fear from anxiety. This distinction is habitually based on the object that induces the emotion: if the object is concrete we would to refer to fear, if the object is vague, poorly defined or even unidentifiable, we would rather refer to anxiety (fear without object). But other levels can also be taken into account (cf. table 1). One of the major points evoked in favor of this distinction is the fact that fear constitutes a basic emotion, while anxiety cannot strictly be considered to be a pure emotion (Lang, 1984). Anxiety appears indeed rather like an indistinct affective state, mixed with fear, but also sadness, anger, or even interest or a feeling of challenge. What seems to make anxiety different from other diffuse affective states such as depression, happiness or shame, essentially lies in two key elements: 1) a certain unpredictability of the feared situation (future), 2) a lack of potential control when facing probable negative events (Barlow, 1988). Every preoccupation is of course focused on the feared situation that may happen: a state of anxious apprehension describes this phenomenon. But a vicious circle can easily set in: the more unpredictable the feared situation proves to be for the person, the more uncontrollable it appears to him, and finally the greater the intensity of preoccupations and anxiety he lives. This state of anxious apprehension develops in pathological anxiety.

Table 1. Classical theoretical distinction between fear and anxiety (according to Barlow, 1988 and Rachman, 1998)

Fear	Anxiety
Concrete object: rational and logical link (shared by everyone) between threat and fear	Source poorly defined, vague: link not clear (not shared by many) between object and anxiety
Limited episode well defined in time	Prolonged duration, persistence, beginning and end not clearly defined
Degree of emergency, imminence of facing a direct and concrete threat	Vigilance, more or less permanent apprehension of future aversive events that are unpredictable and uncontrollable
Physical expression: preparation to act (paralysis, flight or attack)	Cognitive expression: preoccupation, hesitation
Attention directed toward the threat	Attention directed toward oneself
Most extreme expression: panic	Most extreme expression: generalized anxiety

Following Barlow's model (1988), one could conclude that panic represents the pathological expression of fear, and that pathological anxiety (for example generalized anxiety) is the pathological clinical manifestation of anxious apprehension states. However, in clinical practice this distinction between fear and anxiety is not always very easy to do, and doesn't prove to be very useful (Rachman, 1998). In fact fear and anxiety do not appear distinct in the patients' eyes, especially when both states are combined with other psychological symptoms, and furthermore, whether we're dealing with well defined fears or with more vague anxious states does not take on a cardinal importance, since in both cases the therapeutic interventions are fundamentally the same.

2.2. Anxiety Disorders in Psychiatry

The two internationally most employed classifications (ICD-10 and DSM-IV) propose a list of anxiety disorders (American Psychiatric Association, 1994; World Health Organization, 1992). These classifications are supposed to be atheoretical and essentially based on the phenomenology of these disorders. They describe a certain number of syndromes which roughly correspond to the different groups of objects that produce anxiety and to the various manifestations of this emotional state. This is probably the reason why these lists are very similar (cf. table 2). One can however observe some differences between both lists. Firstly, anxiety disorders are classified in the ICD-10 among neurotic disorders (F40) that also include disorders induced by stress factors and somatoform disorders, while in the DSM-IV they are grouped in one unique category. Secondly, the ICD-10 classification divides anxiety disorders in a) phobias, b) other anxiety disorders, c) obsessive-compulsive disorders and d) reactions to stress factors. The American manual does not propose such a sub-classification and prefers to make a simple list of disorders, without any grouping and includes moreover anxiety disorders due to a somatic affection or due to the consumption of substances (which are classed in a completely different heading in the ICD-10). Lastly, let's cite that these two systems separate anxiety disorders from hypochondria. Hypochondria, which is the fear of illnesses (fear to become ill or to have an undiagnosed serious illness) is found in each manual in the section dedicated to somatoform disorders, even if anxiety plays a central role in the clinical picture. In the DSM-IV this section is completely separated from the anxiety disorders section, while in the ICD-10 it classed under the heading including all neurotic disorders (along with the anxiety disorders).

Table 2. Classifications of anxiety disorders according to ICD-10 and DSM-IV

ICD-10	DSM-IV
Phobic anxiety disorders	
Agoraphobia	Agoraphobia without history of panic disorder
Social phobias	Social phobia
Specific phobias	Specific phobias
Other anxiety disorders	
Panic disorder	Panic disorder without agoraphobia
	Panic disorder with agoraphobia
Generalized anxiety disorder	Generalized anxiety disorder
Mixed anxiety and depressive disorder	
Other mixed anxiety disorders	
Other specified anxiety disorders	Anxiety disorder not otherwise specified
Anxiety disorder unspecified	
Obsessive-compulsive disorder (OCD)	
Predominantly obsessional thoughts or ruminations	Obsessive-compulsive disorder
Predominantly compulsive acts	
OCD mixed form with obsessional thoughts and compulsive acts	
Other obsessive-compulsive disorders	
Obsessive-compulsive disorder, unspecified	
Reaction to severe stress and adjustment disorders	
Acute stress reaction	Acute Stress Disorder
Post-traumatic stress disorder	Post-traumatic stress disorder
Adjustment disorders	
Other reactions to severe stress	
Reaction to severe stress, unspecified	
	Anxiety disorder due to a general medical condition
	Substance Induced Anxiety Disorder
Somatoform disorders	*Somatoform disorders*
F45.2 Hypochondrial disorders	Hypochondriasis

Panic disorder is the repetition of well circumscribed episodes characterized by the sudden presence of fear or terror. The disorder is considered serious when more than four panic attacks occur in one month. Panic often happens unpredictably and is associated with physical symptoms such as pounding heart (palpitations), dizziness, muscle tension, tightness in the chest, choking or a feeling of smothering, sweating, trembling, dry mouth, hot or cold flushes, nausea, blurred vision and "jelly legs" (Andrews, Creamer, Crino, Hunt, Lampe and Page, 2003). Panic attacks are by definition frightening experiences that seem strange and abnormal. Because of the intensity of its physical symptoms, panic is habitually accompanied by ideas of collapsing, dying, losing control or becoming crazy. Some people develop a fear of panic: they tend to restrict their activities and to avoid all places where a panic attack is likely occur. Agoraphobia develops then upon the false premise the person has in mind that his panic is provoked by certain situations (restaurants, cinemas, crowded areas, etc.). Panic and agoraphobia seem therefore to be in a continuum where, after the first experiences of intense fear, people tend to avoid them by limiting their lives to areas of security (Andrews et al., 2003). It is not rare that people explain their agoraphobia indicating that they dread more the judgements of others, if they undergo a panic attack, than the fear itself or its somatic consequences. The social consequences of anxiety appear in this case as the crux of the problem: the nature or object of anxiety is social, and it seems relevant here to take into account the differential diagnosis with social phobia.

Social phobia is a strong persisting fear occurring repeatedly in social situations where social performances are required, such as speaking, giving one's own opinions, defending one's rights, making criticisms, demonstrating an exercise, eating with an important person, etc. Feelings of awkwardness, impression to be criticized by others and fear of losing one's own personal value often accompany theses situations and make them extremely unpleasant for the person. Somet«Ges the contact with others is so aversive that panic attacks and agoraphobic avoidance can develop. Panic and avoidance are clearly related to social situations and limited to them, so that diagnoses of panic and/or agoraphobia are not used.

Generalized anxiety disorder is characterized by excessive worry that is continually present during at least 6 months. Preoccupations concern several domains of daily life (work, finances, health, children, etc.) and can virtually touch upon every minor decision or activity the person has to take and to begin. Physical symptoms are present, but with less intensity than in panic: motor tension (restlessness, trembling or muscle tension, headaches, gastric disturbances) and over-excitement (with irritability and difficulties concentrating) and are more prominent than autonomic symptoms (Brown, Marten, and Barlow, 1995; Marten, Brown, Barlow, Borkovec, Shear, and Lydiard, 1993). It is also important to take note that diagnostic rules for DSM-IV and ICD-10 are not identical: by DSM-IV standards, the autonomic symptoms are excluded from the list of physical symptoms, while the ICD-10 requires the presence of an autonomic over-activity for the diagnosis of this disorder.

Post-traumatic stress disorder consists in a prolonged anxious reaction in response to an extremely threatening or catastrophic event. Distress in such situations is normal, but in post-traumatic stress disorder, recovery from the distressing response does not occur. So during weeks, months and even years after the trauma, anxiety and other pathological symptoms can repeatedly occur, handicapping the person in his daily life, and sometimes having extremely heavy consequences on work, relationships and psychological health. Three types of symptoms are habitually described for this syndrome (Andrews et al., 2003): 1) intrusive symptoms such as distressing memories or images of the traumatic event, nightmares, flashbacks where the person relives the incident, and an emotional disruption when reminded of the event; 2) avoidance symptoms consisting in more or less conscious efforts to forget and to escape any reminders of the event, for example gaps in memory, suppressing thoughts about the event, avoiding conversations, places or activities that can remind the person of the event (in serious cases, this avoidance can lead to emotional distance with others and lost of interest in normal activities); 3) over-stimulation symptoms such as the persistence of a state of hypervigilance, sleep disturbances, difficulties in concentrating or irritability. Depression, guilt, consumption of alcohol and drugs are also often present as related problems to PTSD, but the central feature of the pathology is really the incapacity to integrate the fear and horror experience with the existing view of oneself and the world, with a sort of imprisonment in past painful memories.

Obsessive-compulsive disorder is characterized essentially by obsessions and/or compulsions. Obsessive thoughts are ideas, representations or impulsions that repeatedly invade the person's conscience and induce feelings of distress. They are uncontrollable and against the person's will. They touch upon themes such as violence (harm to self or others), obscenity, contamination (being contaminated or being an agent of contamination), religion (blasphemy), etc. Compared to delusions, obsessions are recognized by the person as products of his own mind and are simultaneously criticized as being senseless. Sometimes however obsessions can be overvalued and considered as if they were part of reality. Compulsive behavior (for example: hand washing, sorting, counting, verification) is repetitive and often ritualized activities that respond to a persistent need or urge to act in this particular way, in order to neutralize obsessions or to decrease the discomfort provoked by a situation or a thought. Rituals serve also a preventive function: verifications for example permit, in the individual's mind, to prevent accidents, fire, fatal errors, etc. If the patient is impeded to perform his obsessions and rituals, anxiety and discomfort increase, which can sometimes lead to aggressive behaviors. Obsessive-compulsive patients often become progressively "tyrants" in their families, where all members have to submit to the increasing number of rituals and rules imposed on them by a patient more and more invaded by his fears (for example, interdiction to sit on the sofas, obligation to change clothes when entering the apartment, impossibility to use the phone without having washed one's hands with soap, etc.).

Flow charts can be used in the diagnostic process. They allow to define each syndrome, in comparison with others. They aid the therapist to identify the elements that are similar in all pathologies and the ones that reveal themselves different from one pathology to another (see for example American Psychiatric Association, 1994). Let us not forget that it is also possible that a person can suffer simultaneously from several anxiety disorders. Guidelines, such as the one depicted in figure 1, represent practical ways to proceed in the diagnostic process. For example, one can ask a person first of all if he has gone through episodes of intense panic. If the answer is positive, the diagnosis of panic disorder must be considered and the existence of agoraphobia must be investigated. If the response is negative, one has to verify the existence of a generalized anxiety disorder. Next, one must exclude or include the presence of social phobia, specific phobia or post-traumatic stress disorder by asking the person to detail the contents of their fears. In every case, investigation necessitates the examination of possible organic or substance abuse that could explain anxiety.

Directive and semi-directive structured interviews exist that permit to elaborate in a rigorous and systematic manner the general psychiatric diagnosis or, more specifically, the diagnosis only for anxiety disorders (Brown, DiNardo, and Barlow, 1994; National Institute of Mental Health Molecular Genetics Initiative, 1992; Robins et al., 2000; World Health Organization, 1993).

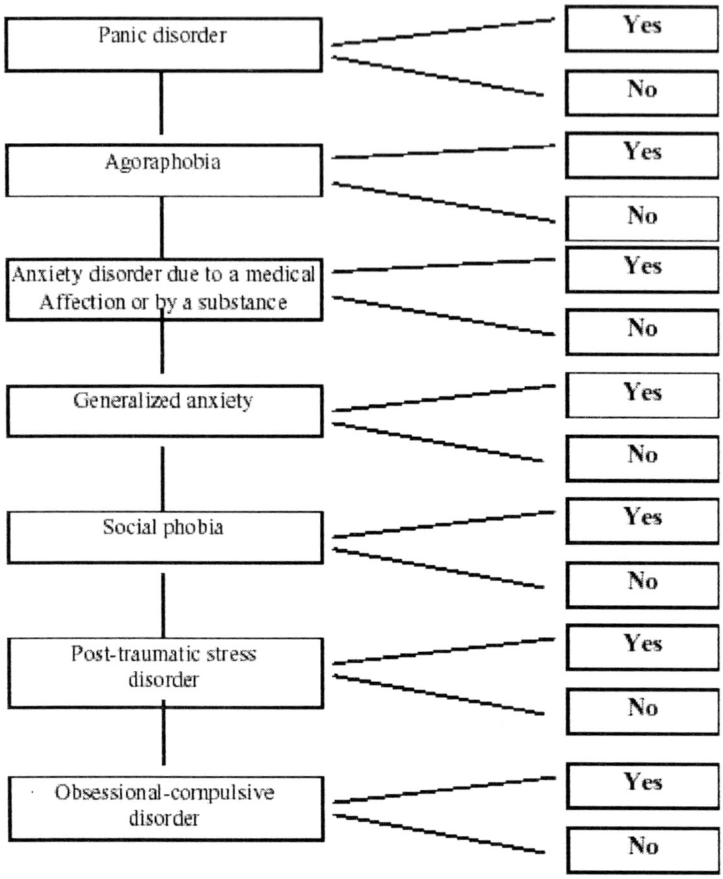

Figure 1. Anxiety disorders investigation guideline

3. The Cognitive-Behavioral Model of Fear

The cognitive and behavioral model is essentially based on current scientific knowledge about psychological disorders, integrating results principally coming from neurosciences and experimental psychology. At its origin, this model was based on the learning paradigm, but has been progressively completed by adding other paradigms such as those coming from the cognitive sciences (for example information processing models), studies on emotions, social psychology, neurobiology and neuropsychology. This model also has a clinical counterpart, offering methods of problem analysis and treatment derived from the conclusions of scientific research. These clinical methods of conceptualization and treatment of anxiety disorders vary from a syndrome to another, but are fundamentally the same. What follows is a brief presentation of this basic general approach.

3.1. Cognitive Behavioral Analysis

The cognitive behavioral approach is founded on the functional analysis of psychological problems (Kanfer and Saslow, 1969; Kanfer and Schefft, 1988). This analysis is based on the following key elements: 1) the choice of a pathological behavior (problem), 2) the identification of the external or internal stimuli preceding (and associated with) the problematic behavior (antecedents), 2) the precise description of the behavior at different phenomenological levels (behavior: cognitive, physiological, affective and motor aspects), 3) the observation of consequences following the behavior (positive/negative, immediate and delayed consequences), 4) the estimation of the degree of contingency between antecedents, behavior and consequences, 5) the analysis of the impact of the individual's mental and physical state on this contingency (for example a woman, when she is tired, will perhaps react more rapidly and more frequently to a particular fear stimulus than when she is fit). The SORCK model proposed by Kanfer (Kanfer and Saslow, 1969; Kanfer and Schefft, 1988), represents a classical way to illustrate with simple categories these basic elements of a functional analysis of a behavior (see figure 2).

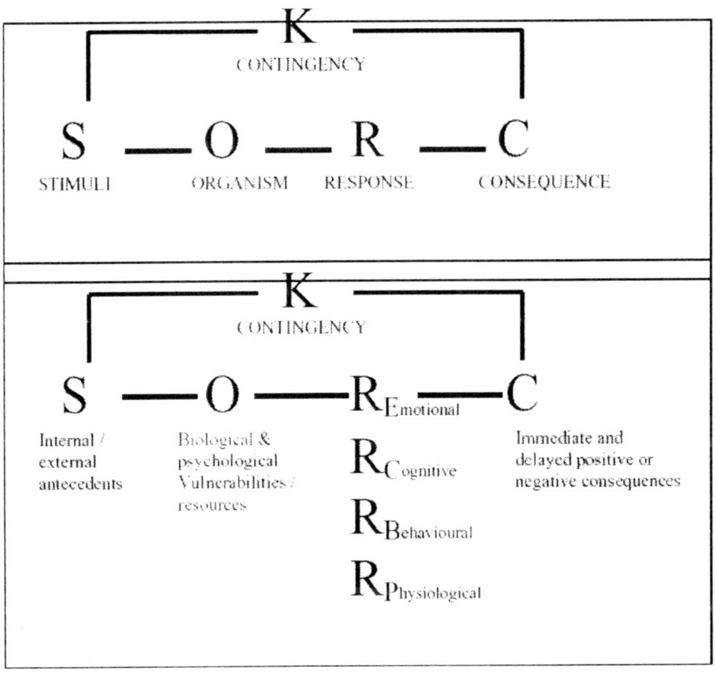

Figure 2. The SORCK model for behavioral functional analysis

The first step of the functional analysis (S in the SORCK model) is the identification of the antecedent stimuli. Stimuli are all the elements of a situation that can set off a particular reaction. In the case of anxiety, the stimuli are all the objects that produce a person's fear or worry. In a given situation, there are indeed particular stimuli that are specifically associated with the fear reaction, and other elements, in the same context, that don't induce a fear reaction and that are therefore neutral. The cognitive behavior therapist's task is to discover with his patient what are these particular fear stimuli.

The second step concerns the description of the psychological problem in behavioral terms (R in the SORCK model). This description gathers observations made at various levels. For example, the affective reaction called fear (emotional level) often represents the starting point for a clinical description. But this labeling is not sufficient. The therapist must identify the physical and physiological characteristics of anxiety (somatic or physiological level): respiratory problems, abdominal pain, shoulder tension, etc. He must also examine thoughts concomitant with these reactions (cognitive level): "Its unbearable.", "I'll never make it.", "Here we go, it's happening again! It's horrible! I have to get out of here right away.", etc. Finally motor aspects of behavior are also described, trying to answer this basic interrogation: what does the person do in this situation? Most of the time we will see a reaction of flight from the feared situation or avoidance of confronting himself to this situation (avoidance is habitually present when fear precedes the "danger" itself, that is in the case of anticipatory fears). Other motor behaviors can be attempts to relax, the taking of sedative medication, a phone call to a spouse or companion, a pause in activity, alcohol consumption, etc. The simple emotional label of "fear" can therefore conceal a very large number of different somatic-cognitive-behavioral profiles that this phenomenological description can bring more clearly into the picture.

The third step of this analysis considers the consequences of the behavior itself (C in the SORCK model). On a very short-term basis, the result usually turns out positive: the escape behavior produces a feeling of relief. But the long-term consequences become less advantageous: handicap and social withdrawal (for example agoraphobic persons become isolated and no longer leave their houses alone), the renouncement of a professional activity, marital conflicts, etc. These consequences frequently drive the person to consult a specialist, sometimes after having spent years or decades organizing their lives around their anxiety. Often specialized help is not even sought (Pollard, Henderson, Frank, and Margolis, 1989).

The last two steps of the functional analysis concern: 1) the contingency between the behavioral and the environmental aspects of the problem and 2) the link between the person's global mental and physical state and the frequency and intensity of his problematic behavior (understood in the sense of biological and psychological vulnerabilities). Contingency represents the strength of the association between stimuli, responses and their consequences (K in the SORCK model). Certain stimuli or configurations of stimuli can systematically induce intense fear, while other stimuli provoke this emotion only one out of ten times and at lesser intensities. A big German Shepherd without a leash, barking and chasing after a person will certainly set off in this person a reaction of intense fear, even more if he suffers from dog phobia. Other stimuli connected to dogs will however provoke in the same individual only moderate anxious responses: for example a picture of a dog, a Dachshund on a leash, or a Cocker spaniel eating out of his dish. In the same way, contingency can concern the link between response and consequence. Certain behaviors won't systematically reduce anxiety: for example an attempt at relaxation exercises won't always be totally or even partially effective. In obsessive compulsive disorders, it is not rare that executing the rituals (for example washing one's hands in order to destroy bacterium or to eliminate any trace of filthiness) results in more anxiety than before, as if the person fell in a trap where the behavior that previously relieved anxiety now increases it. The degree of the person's vulnerability (for example state of fatigue, stress, menstruations, personality traits, etc.) indicates that he can be more or less fragile: in a state of vulnerability, less or less intense stimuli can generate fear and have the same effect as stimuli that are a priori more fear inducing (Connor-Smith and Compas, 2002; Friedman, Clark, and Gershon, 1992). This is due to the fact that stress and anxiety are intimately linked (Friedman et al., 1992; Gray, 1991; Robinson, Corbett, and Spurlock, 1996). Vulnerability, in the broad sense of the term, can be a stable biological or psychological trait (indicated by biological or psychological markers) as well as a transient state depending on a particular person's circumstances which in turn can be induced or controlled or not by him (stress induced by a major life event, consumption of coffee or alcohol, etc.). Personal resources represent another form of a stable trait or transient state that can influence the degree of contingency between the antecedents, the behaviors and their consequences (for example a weak tendency to be physically stimulated, coping resources in the face of problems, capacity to seek external help, etc.). These variables determine whether a person will be more or less able to manage their stressful situations. Theses resources and vulnerability states/traits are represented by the organism variable in the SORCK model (O).

The SORCK model leads the therapist to the discovery and precise observation of all the active elements that can influence the behavioral problem under analysis. This model should allow the understanding and even the prediction of anxiety responses in the various situations the patient can go through. The therapist will also be able to verify the role of the immediate and delayed consequences of the various responses the person has when facing his anxiety problem. It appears evident enough that the more meticulous the analysis is, the better the prediction will turn out to be. Nevertheless, it is rarely necessary to attain a very high degree of precision in order to start a treatment. Two to four hours prove habitually to be sufficient to formulate a hypothesis derived from the functional analysis of the patient and this provides the tools that can be used to propose a treatment plan. This hypothesis will be then adapted and corrected according to the newbandata and clinical observations gathered during the treatment. If necessary, this hypothesis can be totally reassessed in the light of new important information or events, and the treatment consequently adjusted. The therapeutic process functions as a constant adaptation of the treatment procedures to the hypothesis elaborated to explain the clinical data.

3.2. The Cognitive-Behavioral Model of Anxiety

In order to explain its origin and its development, the cognitive-behavioral model of anxiety calls upon basic psychological processes. The learning paradigm is principally used through conditioning models (classical-associative and operant conditioning), cognitive information processing models, and the social cognitive learning model.

Historically, the associative learning model was the first explored in studying anxiety. According to this model, fear and phobias often result from the association between a neutral stimulus and one or more stimuli that automatically produced an initial reaction of fear (for example an aversive stimulus or a situation that is really dangerous). These stimuli that automatically cause fear are called unconditioned stimuli, because they are the source of an uncontrollable reflex response of the organism. The classical or associative conditioning links one or more neutral stimuli to these unconditional stimuli that induce the automatic reaction of fear. Neutral stimuli then become conditioned stimuli, because they can now produce fear reactions by themselves, without the presentation of an unconditioned fear stimulus. In this case, fear is a learned response that can be set off automatically by one or more conditioned stimuli that have become themselves fear inducing (Barlow, 1988; Gray, 1991; Rachman, 1978). For example, imagine that just after a small painful bite, a young child develops a fear of goats. He refuses now to pet them while before the incident he indulged in this activity with enthusiasm. Any sudden movements of the animal's head will make him start, because these movements are associated with the painful bite.

We know today that the conditioning of fear is particularly resistant and efficient: sometimes only one association is enough to create a conditioning (Rescorla, 1988). For example, tainted food can cause already after a first experience a definitive aversive reaction, which can be extremely difficult to cancel out: the same food, but fresh, wouldn't even be tasted. Moreover, conditioning can take place even when the two stimuli (the neutral and the unconditional) don't take place at the same time (Mackintosh, 1983). The conditioning seems to appear later after the association between a fear reaction and a neutral stimulus. Let's imagine that the goat's bite is not immediately followed by fear in the child, who, after a short period of crying, continues to pet other goats which have not bitten him. However, after a more or less brief passage of time, the child associates "goat" and "bite" and develops a fear of goats in general (in order to avoid the pain, thinking for example that all goats are in reality unpredictable in their movements). New theories show that even classical conditioning is not a simple reflex reaction: a complex internal information process selectively associates physiological and affective reactions with particular stimuli that are most likely not chosen in a random manner. The conditioning helps to inform the individual about the probable causes of different positive or negative reactions he has had. In this sense conditioning appears as a "mechanical" process as well as a cognitive one (Bandura, 1977; Mackintosh, 1983) that allows the organism to predict his environment (physical and interpersonal) and to adjust consequently its own reactions.

The operant conditioning hypothesis about fear is based on escape/avoidance behavior. This particular behavior reinforces the fear reaction by relieving the subject of his negative consequences (unpleasantness of the negative emotion). This process is called negative reinforcement, because the escape behavior allows the subject to reduce the negative consequences of fear (Mowrer, 1960, Salkovskis, Clark, Hackmann, Wells, and Gelder, 1999). Indeed, escape or avoidance behaviors are central in the maintenance process of anxiety and the development of anxiety disorders. However they can't explain their origin, that is they are not the causes of fear and anxiety. Avoiding or escaping any threat appears completely natural and logical (Gray, 1991): the child will no longer pet the biting goat (avoidance), he will pull his hand away when a goat suddenly moves his head (escape). But by systematically pulling his hand away, the child no longer has the possibility to realize that movements of the goat's head do not always mean that he'll be bitten; on the contrary he will congratulate himself for having escaped from the bite (even if this isn't really true) and learn nothing else than the escape behavior, which will be then reinforced. As he avoids the so called danger, the individual can no longer convince himself that there isn't any real danger. He gets himself into a position where it is for him impossible to learn a new way to deal with the situation (in the present case: how to pet a goat without being bitten!). If the goat example seems a little humorous, analogous situations with a snake (even a non-poisonous one), an hairy spider, an angry and domineering boss, or even the example of a man with a young beautiful woman (or a woman with an handsome young man) are surely much easier to identify with for the reader.

In summary, two forms of conditioning seem to play a key role in the learning of an anxiety disorder: 1) a classical conditioning where neutral stimuli become fear through association with unconditioned stimuli that automatically set off fear; 2) an operant conditioning where avoidance and escape behaviors are reinforced and repeated because they reduce the fear (but without giving the possibility to eliminate it completely). This rather rudimentary model, known as the two factors model (Mowrer, 1960), represents the first historical step in the cognitive-behavioral conceptualization of anxiety disorders. Even though it's dated, it hasn't lost all its pertinence and still constitutes a simple way to explain anxiety problems (Rachman, 1998).

Current models are more complex and use also knowledge derived from cognitive psychology. The role of cognitions has been particularly underlined and studied. In fact the study of cognitions has allowed to understand clinical cases and situations where the conditioning models have proved to be rather limited and unsatisfactory. Cognitive models argue that emotion is mediated by cognition, and that in a given situation the nature of a person's thoughts determines his emotional feelings (Beck and Emery, 1985; Salkovskis, 1996). Beck's model constitutes a key reference for the general cognitive conceptualization of psychiatric disorders (Beck, Rush, Shaw, and Emery, 1979). This author proposes to differentiate beliefs or schemas from automatic thoughts. Schemas (or beliefs) represent a sort of interpretative reality filter that can be activated or not in certain situations. When it's activated, a schema will promote the production of thoughts congruent with it (in competition with alternative thoughts which could challenge it). These thoughts are called "automatic" because the individual can hardly control them: they furnish a first and immediate interpretation of reality which gives a particular sense to it. These automatic thoughts can next colour the emotional experience in a positive or a negative way depending on their contents. It is actually hard to know if thoughts have preceded emotions or not; but in any case, their mutual relationships and the parallelism in the contents are always quite obvious: fear is very often related to threatening thoughts, sadness or depression can accompany gloomy and pessimistic thoughts. Automatic thoughts can often take an absolute and nuance-deprived character. Their imperative, timeless and generalizing aspects (thoughts are applied to any circumstance, without any consideration of a situation's particularity), often make up veritable cognitive tyrants against whom it is frequently very difficult to resist.

Beck's work demonstrates that anxious and depressive automatic thoughts are distorted views of reality: they don't resist to logical analysis. The premise of cognitive therapy is then to get the patients to progressively realize that they suffer because they do not correctly treat information received from their environments (when for example they consider as threatening something which is actually innocuous). Challenging theses cognitive distortions can bring new thoughts about the feared situations and favourably influence their anxiety. Table 3 synthesizes the habitual cognitive distortions observed in therapy by anxious and depressive patients. The reader will be aware of the importance of the words themselves used or of the subtle deviations from a pure logical analysis of a situation (in the anticipations, inferences, pseudo-logical conclusions, etc. made by the patients). Cognitive distortions are a normal part of human thinking. They are deeply discussed in therapy only because certain are hypothesized to have lead to emotional disorders. The idea is not to suppress all forms of cognitive distortions but to reduce the impact of the ones that are directly connected to psychological disorders.

Beck theorizes that behind automatic thoughts, there exists a great variety in beliefs and schemas. These schemas are progressively constructed during childhood. They reflect an individual's vision of the world and of himself, which has been forged through his developmental history, the influences of his surroundings, his education and his more or less traumatizing life events (Ingram, Miranda, and Segal, 1998). Beliefs explain why the automatic thoughts are provoking thoughts. According to their types of beliefs, the world will be considered as threatening and dangerous, the self as vulnerable and the future as unpredictable and incontrollable by subjects suffering from anxiety disorders (Beck and Emery, 1985). In comparison a depression-provoking schema will lead the person to interpret his world as negative, without worth, himself as useless and helpless, and his future as lost or without hope (Blackburn and Davidson, 1990). If cognitive schemas don't change even after psychological treatment, they constitute one of the aspects of the individual's vulnerability towards anxiety or depression (Ingram et al., 1998; Rachman, 1998).

Table 3. Definitions and examples of the most frequent cognitive distortions (Blackburn, 1992; Blackburn and Davidson, 1990)

Cognitive distortion	Definition	Example
Selective abstraction	To consider only a part of reality to give meaning to a situation. To draw a conclusion only from one or two details (often of poor significance)	Surprised by a difficult question, an orator says to himself " I must really be a bad speaker; he will tell to all others that I'm a stupid man. Then everyone will make fun of me ".
Arbitrary inference	To make conclusions without proof or even to insist upon a conclusion in the presence of contradicting facts	" My boss didn't say anything about my being late with Mr Muller's file, I'm sure he's going to fire me "
Overgeneralisation	To apply one unique form of reasoning for all possible situations.	" Everyone thinks I'm stupid " " All dogs bite " " Every physical symptom announces a sudden and serious illness "
Minimisation or maximalisation	To evaluate in an erroneous way the intensity or the importance of a reaction/event (exaggeration of suffering and minimalization of success).	" I can't stand it " " Anyone can do what I did "
Personalization	To refer independent events only to oneself; to attribute the cause of an event only to oneself.	" The new supervisor hasn't talked to me yet, I must not be smart enough for her. " " It's my fault if ... "
Dichotomic thought	To interpret situations only in extreme categories (black or white, all or nothing, good or bad) without any possibility of a shade of grey between two opposites	" Either I'm a courageous man who can confront any dangerous situation, or I'm a looser and a coward. " " Either I have success with this woman, or I'll never attract any woman . "

Other forms of cognitions and cognitive processes have also been studied in anxiety disorders. One of them is self-efficacy beliefs, a sort of expectation, that Bandura (1986) conceptualized in his social cognitive model of human behavior. Self-efficacy beliefs reveal the individuals' perception of their capabilities to perform effectively and to achieve specific results. Self-efficacy is a cognition that precedes action, because it influences the choice of an individual to begin or not a particular activity or behavior. If the person thinks 1) that the behavior he wants to adopt will help him to achieve his desired goals (outcome expectations) and 2) that he's able to perform effectively this behavior (personal competence or self-confidence), then he will adopt it. The answers to both questions are naturally dependent on the pursued goals and the current and particular context where the person is (affective state, social and environmental conditions, past history, etc.). But if the individual responds negatively to one of these two questions, the probability that he doesn't behave in this way increases.

According to Bandura's (1986) social cognitive theory, self-efficacy is a key element of to motivation. It is a part of a self system that enables to exercise self-regulation of behaviors, thoughts and feelings. Through this self control system individuals possess the capability to influence their own thoughts and actions. Self-efficacy beliefs influence these motivational and self-regulatory processes in several ways: a) by acting on the choices to do something and to pursue this action, b) by determining how much effort will be expended on an activity, c) by deciding how long an effort will be persevered when obstacles appear. Efficacy beliefs also influence the amount of stress experienced by individuals as they engage in a task. Strong self-efficacy beliefs clearly enhance feelings of personal accomplishment and well-being. On the other hand, people with low self-efficacy may believe that things are more difficult than they really are; a belief that fosters stress and feelings of helplessness. In the case of anxiety, this model is particularly useful to predict if a person will expose himself to his proper fears, and to what extent he will agree to be confronted with his anxiety-provoking situations (Bandura, 1988).

Another important cognitive aspect reported in anxiety concerns the attentional processes. It seems in fact that one can observe during anxious episodes a double movement of attention: 1) a global scanning in search of threatening elements in the environment (vigilance or hypervigilance), 2) during the experience of fear itself, a focalization on what is internally felt (attentional self-focus). These movements of attention favor the development of fear and even panic. Self-focused attention appears indeed as an important maintaining factor in anxiety disorders because it increases access to negative thoughts and feelings, interferes with performance, and prevents the individual from observing external information that might disconfirm his or her fears (Clark and Wells, 1995).

Hypervigilance, by maintaining the organism prepared for danger, favours physiological excitation and cognitive stress. Cognitively, the individual directs his attention toward all potential threats (those of course that depend on his own cognitive schemas, personal phobias, and negative expectations); physiologically his organism is in a state of tension necessary for immediate and rapid action. This state of hypervigilance probably results from a cognitive fear schema (for example: the world is dangerous and I'm vulnerable to any possible attack), as we've seen before in Beck's model. Barlow (1988) proposes to call this type of schema an apprehensive hypervalent cognitive schema which roughly corresponds to the predisposition of an individual to detect in a given situation all sources of negative affect, in order to avoid it. It appears clearly that in this state of cognitive and physiological tension, the occurence of a stress or anxious reaction becomes more probable even in less demanding contexts.

When a stress reaction is started, the focalization on one's internal experience increases this reaction through the salience of perception. Because the person is more concentrated on what's internally happening than on the outside world or on the activity that has to be accomplished, he will be highly receptive to his internal stimuli: consequently the emotional experience is intensified and the habituation to fear stimuli reduced (Scheier, Carver, and Matthews, 1983). Furthermore, the direct consequence of this dysfunction in attention is a possible reduction in the performance quality during a task, or even its failure: the individual feels paralysed by emotion, he can't find his words, he doesn't remember even obvious things, he can no longer organize or plan out his activity, simple gestures are executed awkwardly, etc. This decline in performance troubles in turn the person who will associate the situation with his anxiety and failure or incompetence. From now on he will fear the return of this emotion that will be equal to him as a return of incompetence. On a long term basis, individuals can abandon their activities because they are afraid of being invaded by anxiety when performing.

Conceptualizations of anxiety have varied and been refined over time. Researchers have elaborated more and more complete models, or have orientated themselves towards different and new or poorly investigated aspects of these disorders. We have described here three or four various learning paradigms and cognitive models which were applied to anxiety. From these multiple visions it is now central to try to find out the essential points that might constitute a global psychological model of anxiety disorders as a basis for the explanations given to patients or to the general public.

1. We can consider fear and anxiety as alarm reactions that are more or less intense. Fear's function is to warn the individual of a danger, and to prepare the organism to affront it or to flee. Because of this, fear is a negative reaction: it is perceived as unpleasant for the individual, and therefore avoided. These alarms can be justified (in front of real danger) or not (in phobias). In this last case, we talk of false alarms, because they don't warn of real dangers. Real or false alarms aren't pathological in themselves. Pathology derives from the fact that these alarms are inadequately and repetitively set off in non threatening situations.
2. People apparently show specific individual predispositions to develop anxious reactions (physiological vulnerability or higher sensitivity to stress, cognitive vulnerability in the form of fear cognitive schemas). According to the "diathesis-stress" model the interaction between personal vulnerability and stress factors can favour the development of anxiety disorders, particularly in contexts when the subject's capacities of adaptation and stress management are overwhelmed.
3. Anxiety disorders most likely result from learning. Initial alarms (real or false) become learned alarms that inappropriately occur in innocuous situations. The origin of the disorder is not always all that clear. One can suppose in some cases that a naturally phobogenic stimulus has favored a conditioning: stimuli that are associated to those that cause the initial reaction of fear can in turn become fear. However it is not always easy to find out what the initial conditioning was and in what context it appeared. In any case, because of the negative value of anxious affect, the individual rapidly learns the behaviors that relieve him from anxiety.

These are essentially escape (flight) or avoidance. They are reinforced by their positive consequences on a short term basis (relief from anxiety), but they have a negative effect on a long term basis. Avoidance actually favours the maintaining of anxiety in three ways: 1) it blocks the processes of natural habituation to fear stimuli and to physiological reactions of anxiety, because each time the stimuli are perceived and anxiety is felt, the whole process is stopped by the escape behavior which brutally interrupts the negative emotion, 2) it doesn't permit the individual to have the concrete experience that the feared situation doesn't contain any real danger, and to thusly modify his internal representations and interpretations, 3) it impedes the development of anxiety management strategies that are more constructive and less handicapping. Therefore flight and avoidance are at the same time natural and automatic behaviors in the face of anxiety, but also big contributors to the processes that maintain anxiety as a pathological state.

4. Different cognitive processes mediate anxiety reactions and can install a vicious cycle of anxious apprehension (Barlow, 1988). The existence of these processes permits to distinguish normal anxiety (where they are absent) from pathological anxiety. Three types of cognition are implied: 1) attentional processes, 2) outcome and self-efficacy expectancies, 3) cognitive schemas and automatic thoughts.

At the attentional level, we first observe hypervigilance in people suffering from anxiety disorders. These subjects are in a state of anxious apprehension that is more or less permanent. Hypervigilance is particularly present in situations where there's a high probability of occurrence of feared events. Attention is focalized here on the external environment, to detect every probable danger, in order to avoid it or to reduce its impact. But in the case where negative affect is set off, attention is then directed toward the internal experience. This in turn increases emotion even more (which therefore favors the escape behavior!). Moreover, the redirection of attention on the internal experience does not allow good task performances because the attentional resources are no longer allocated to the right place. This results in an effective decrease in the quality of activity that in turn plays a role in the subject's interpretation of the situation (lowering of self-esteem, feeling of loss of control, incapacity to face things, negative expectations, etc.). These movements of attentional processes play therefore a role in the vicious circle of anxiety, Fear of failure nourishing avoidance behaviors (which impede habituation to fear and innocuous feared stimuli) is itself justified by real failures due to fear! If this process is highly adaptive in the case of real danger (where failure can mean se□^{2}ous wounds or death), it becomes pathological in phobias by maintaining the fears rather than by diminishing them.

Hypervigilance is naturally concomitant with anticipative thoughts and negative expectations. Anxious expectations tend in their contents to consider the world as threatening and unpredictable and to see the individual as weak and incapable to deal with his problems or to control the course of events. These characteristics of unforeseeability, personal vulnerability and uncontrollability seem by the way to constitute the specific traits that allow distinguishing anxious individuals from others (Barlow, 1988). With negative self-efficacy and outcome expectancies, the individual will be less inclined to begin courageous attempts to confront his feared situations. That maintains him in an avoidant attitude which doesn't allow the reduction of the anxious apprehension process.

These negative expectations have without a doubt their substrate in thought schemas that are profoundly anchored in man's persona. Schemas are beliefs about oneself and the world that act as interpretative filters of reality. They can be activated or not in certain situations through hypothesized associative processes and neurocognitive nodes in the brain. The activation of such cognitive schemas will in difficult situations produce automatic thoughts that provide the individual with a key to immediate interpretation of what's happening. These thoughts guide him toward the attitude to follow. Unfortunately these interpretations are often biased. They communicate a series of cognitive distortions that end up rendering the person weakly adapted and weakly adaptable. Automatic thoughts, congruent with the underlying cognitive beliefs, tend to exaggerate the severity and the dangerousness of the situation and the person's weaknesses in a way that they negatively color affect.

In summary cognitive, behavioral and physiological processes contribute to the maintaining of anxiety. The adaptive reasons are obvious: a habituation that is too rapid and a disinterest in front of real dangers would quickly drive our species toward extinction. We can therefore affirm that the processes in themselves do not allow to judge if anxiety is pathological or not. Anxiety will be considered pathological when it's maintained by the vicious cycle of anxious apprehension favouring the importunate production of anxious episodes in situations that are not dangerous for the person (Barlow, 1988). Pathology therefore lays more in the contents or objects of anxiety, in the suffering and handicap that's follow, than in the implicated psychological processes, which are in a certain sense normal and adaptive but displaced. Changing anxiety reactions apply then to almost identical methods used to modify any old bad habits! We will briefly review in the next section some of the habitual methods employed in the cognitive behavior therapy of anxiety disorders, without entering in the details and the variants developed specifically for every particular disorder.

4. Methods of Intervention in Cognitive-Behavior Therapies for Anxiety

The different facets of anxiety and the processes that are implicated represent as many entry points for therapeutic intervention. In fact, behavioral and cognitive approaches have provided for therapists a large arsenal of methods that aim to modify one or another aspect of the anxious reaction (cf. table 4). Behavioral interventions focus on flight and avoidance behaviors that they attempt to decrease. They favour the development of alternative coping strategies that don't have the disadvantages of flight or avoidance. Cognitive interventions target automatic thoughts and underlying beliefs, attentional processes, and negative expectations. The goal is to aid the patient to regain a certain degree of control on these cognitive processes and positively modify their role in the vicious circle of anxiety. Interventions on a physical level try to reduce the physiological impact of anxious reactions. If he succeeds, the subject will feel to a lesser degree the physical signals of anxiety. He will consequently concentrate his attention less on them, and therefore will not be overwhelmed by the intensity of his emotional reactions. In general, treatment strategies combine various specific techniques. For example, the emotional reprocessing, which is certainly a central feature of any psychotherapy, is the combination of behavioral and cognitive techniques, because for emotional processing to occur, exposure has to be done with cognitive restructuring that allow the corrective experience necessary for change (Barlow, 1988; Foa and Kozak, 1986; Rachman, 1980). The separation of techniques is relatively artificial; clearly separate categories of interventions are generally made only for pedagogical purposes. In practice the therapists tend to use them conjointly and to integrate them in individualized strategies elaborated for every patient or group of patients.

Table 4. Goals and methods of intervention in behavioral cognitive approach to anxiety

Dimension	Goal of treatment	Possible interventions
Behavior	To eliminate escape and avoidance behaviors	Exposure with response prevention and development of alternative anxiety management strategies (coping strategies)
Affect	To accept the experience of anxiety and to favour the emotional reprocessing of anxiety	Emotional reprocessing: exposure to the full emotional experience (at all levels: behavioral, cognitive and physiological) that allows the learning of corrective information (especially: anxiety will not last indefinitely, the real probability of harm and danger is low, the emotion itself is not unbearable).
Thought	To reorient attention towards the task	Self-instructions (in the hope of regaining control of attentional processes that guide the reorientation towards the task). Learning and use of problem solving techniques.
	To modify expectations of negative self-efficacy	Discussion and reflection about the relevance of the negative expectations; prospective comparisons between expectations and what really happens; experience of success in difficult situations; observation and imitation of successful models. Cognitive restructuration (by Socratic interviewing methods); identification and correction techniques of automatic thoughts ; psychopedagogical intervention.
	To modify automatic fear thoughts and replace them by more realistic ones	Cognitive restructuration through Socratic interviews, evaluation of the relevance and the usefulness of different schemas of thought (intervenes later in treatment).
	To modify the basic cognitive schemas that produce fear automatic thoughts	
Physical	To reduce the physiological intensity of excitation and stress concomitant with the experience of anxiety	Relaxation, breathing exercises, vaso-vagal techniques for reduction of heart rate, biofeedback.

Paradoxically the first goal of cognitive behavior therapy for anxiety is not the total elimination of any anxiety reaction (that would be catastrophic for the individual's survival). It rather proposes a relearning procedure, where the patient will progressively understand his own emotional functioning, accept it and try to master its different aspects. He will learn to isolate the cognitive and behavioral automatisms that maintain anxiety in inadequate contexts. According to Barlow (1988), three targets are essential to the success of anxiety treatments:

1) the modification of action tendencies associated with anxiety (avoidance, escape, but also hypervigilance), 2) the development of a feeling of control towards the environment (in spite of the presence of emotional signs of anxiety: events are not totally out of control, one can do something active to change the current situation), 3) the reorientation of attentional processes towards the task (instead of maintaining a self-focused attention on the internal experience). Other targets or goals of treatment (such as modification of automatic thoughts or reduction of physiological arousal) appear useful but according to this author remain secondary: these aspects modify themselves when the emotional reprocessing has been successfully done.

4.1. Behavioral Interventions

Methods of behavioral intervention have as a goal to reduce or even eliminate avoidance and escape in situations where they shouldn't be present. This is in fact one if not *the* key points in any anxiety therapy. The principal technique of behavioral intervention is exposure with response prevention. Multiple variants have been developed of which the guiding rule is always the same: "anxiety will decrease if you stay in the innocuous feared situation. If you let yourself completely live the anxious reactions that the situation induces, without turning to avoidance or any safety behaviours, this could reassure you without totally convincing you that the situation and its related anxiety are not dangerous and unbearable".

The efficiency of durable exposure has been understood for a long time through processes of cognitive and physiological habituation or extinction of the anxious response. Figure 3 is often presented to patients as a simple explanatory model and as a justification of the regular practice of this technique.

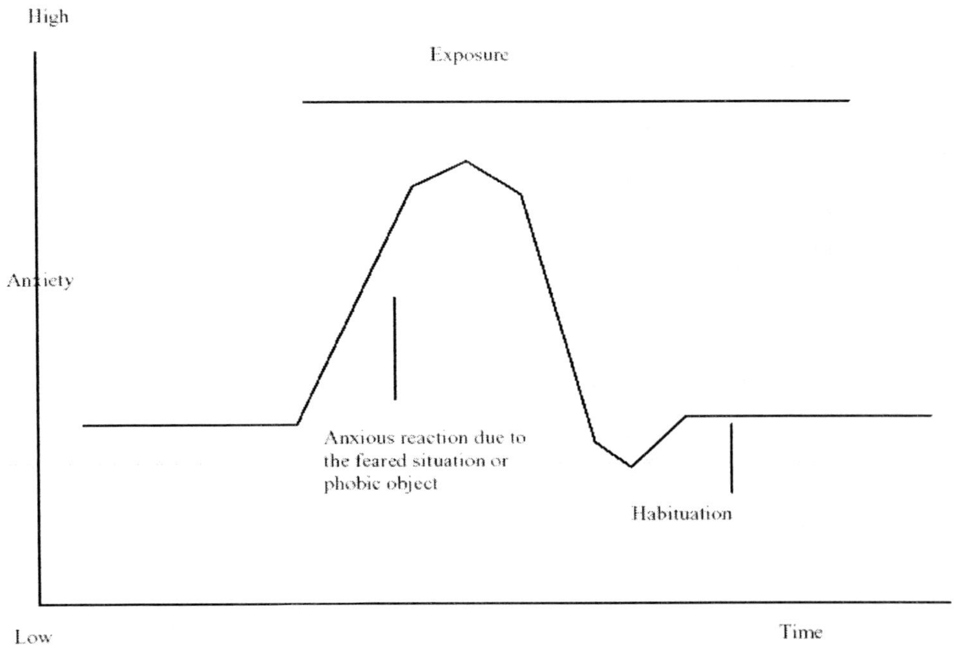

Figure 3. Processes of anxiety and habituation responses in feared situations

The model predicts that if the person fully experiences anxiety, without escaping the situation, without being wounded in any way, and becoming more and more aware that the dangers and other catastrophic scenarios are only the products of his imagination, his emotional reaction will tend to disappear with time. It can take hours before the first panic progressively resolves to become a sensation of weak tension, and only the rehearsal of exposure exercises will provide the necessary confidence to approach with tranquillity that which before produced intense fear. The organism gets used to anxiety evoking stimuli just as someone gets used to the noise of a train that regularly goes by their window, to the point where they don't even hear the express rushing by each hour to the next station. As with the train, feared situations (the noise of the trains) attract attention, but little by little the organism recognizes them automatically, concluding that there is no danger, and no longer directs its attention towards them. After a period of being exposed to feared situations, the individual ends up learning that the negative consequences he feared do not occur. In these conditions, the strength of the link decreases and the stimuli from their anxiety-provoking state return to a sort of neutrality state.

Habituation and extinction are two major facets of the process of anxiety reduction (Barlow, 1988). Habituation refers to the natural reduction of the response's intensity (often measured on a physiological level); it is in relation with biological processes that are controlled on a primary neurological level. Extinction refers to the reduction of the strength of the conditioning when the fear stimuli are not followed by real negative consequences. It is the equivalent of unlearning the link between stimulus and response. In this way, habituation corresponds to a form of exhaustion of the biological response to anxiety, while extinction can happen only if the exposure is not followed by negative consequences (Barlow, 1988). Given this, extinction deals more with cognitive processes while habituation seems rather a physiological phenomenon. With the habituation process, the individual learns that the anxiety response does not indefinitely persist and that it naturally ceases with time, while in extinction he understands that the situation is in reality not dangerous and that therefore the alarm reaction has no reason to be triggered off. A cognitive invalidation of the negative expectations would therefore exist that could mediate the process of anxiety reduction, even if behavioral methods are used as primary therapeutic techniques (Seligman and Johnston, 1973).

Exposure can be gradual or massive, done in imagination or in vivo (Leahy and Holland, 2000; Marks, 1987). Graded exposure is based on a hierarchy of fear stimuli previously established with the patient. It indicates the intensity of the anxiety for each item, ranging from the weakest to the most intense. The person progressively exposes himself to the anxiety-evoking situations, respecting this hierarchy: only when he has successfully mastered the weakly feared items, he then confronts himself with the items that are more delicate to manage. Before he carries out the in-vivo exposure, the person does it in imagination, thinking about the fear stimuli (and not directly confronting them). Once a person is capable of mentally coping without fear with his perilous situations, he will more easily be able to dare to expose himself to the real situations. Massive exposure is a lot more direct and doesn't bother itself with a complicated preparation: the individual is plunged from the beginning into the worst situation for himself and he must face it until habituation occurs. Compared to graded exposure, in vivo massive exposure (flooding) or implosion procedures (massive exposure in imagination) requires more time in the situation, but assuredly shortens the length of therapy. Massive exposure unfortunately presents the major defect of enticing very few patients to adopt it as treatment; the drop out rate in this therapy is significantly higher than the 12% habitually described in graded exposure therapies (Emmelkamp and Wessels, 1975; Jannoun, Munby, Catalan, and Gelder, 1980; Matthews et al., 1976). Furthermore, a brutal change in a person's behavioral habits can directly affect the interactions with the surroundings, bringing the risk of a negative destabilisation for the patient or his family (Himadi et al., 1986; Peter and Hand, 1988). In most cases and in particular with very anxious patients, the therapist will therefore prefer to adopt a progressive strategy, that is maybe slower, but generally more easily accepted.

Exposure treatments are conducted in four steps. The first consists of a socialization to treatment: the patients are informed about the behavioral model of anxiety where the role of escape/avoidance is especially stressed. The rationale of the exposure therapy is clearly explained and the steps of the treatment described. To help more anxious clients to accept this treatment, the preparatory phase can be extended to the learning of some coping strategies (relaxation training, self-instructions, etc.). Clients can in this way feel more confident to entry the exposure phase of the therapy, which induces often great apprehension.

In the second step, patients create with their therapists a hierarchy of items including the major cues that provoke anxiety. Theses cues are ranked from least to most difficult in an anxiety-scale (in 8 or 10 points, from tranquillity to panic). Habitually lists of 10-15 items are generated with the preoccupation that every point of the anxiety scale corresponds with at least one specific item. If the items are ranked either at the bottom or at the top of the scale graded exposure cannot be easily conducted, because it is impossible to program exposure exercises with a real graduation of the difficulty. This work is also an occasion to identify more precisely the various cues that can produce anxiety and sometimes to deepen the understanding of various facets of the disorder. With flooding strategies (massive exposure), a list of fear stimuli is also collected in order to identify all fear cues and to determine what could be a very difficult exposure situation to confront with. The more massive the exposure is, the more time the therapist must dedicate to it: habitually 40 to 120 minutes are sufficient to complete the procedure, but with massive exposure or with some serious cases (such as obsessive-compulsive disorders) durations can be much longer and last more than 4-5 hours. In this case, graded exposures are often preferred both by patients and by therapists (increasing also compliance to the treatment), because they are less difficult to conduct and are also less time consuming; it is however not proved that they are more effective than massive exposures (Fiegenbaum, 1988).

Thirdly an initial exposure is prepared and worked through during a therapy session. This exposure can be an in vivo exposure or an imaginary exposure (depending on the therapeutic strategy negotiated with the patient). In graded exposure, this step begins with an item that is at the bottom of the list, so that the exercise doesn't trigger too much anxiety. The patients have the opportunity here to make a first positive and successful experience in confronting himself with anxiety. Therapist should be aware that, although the first items are perhaps relatively easy to confront with, anxiety symptoms should appear during exposure and the patients should go through this emotional experience without avoiding it or trying to reassure themselves with any safety signals or behaviors. This is the reason why it is often recommended to cease pharmacological treatment before the exposure intervention: clients should not attribute their successes to the anxiolytic drug or other talismans or hidden self-protection measures... For the first exposure to be a successful experiment, patients should have experienced the increase in anxiety and the habituation process where tension and symptoms progressively decrease (if they not completely disappear). Exposure mustn't be terminated before the entire process of habituation has been completed. The risk is then more the result of a sensitization to anxiety with an avoidance strategy than a real habituation/extinction process.

Finally the last step consists of the rehearsal of the exposure exercise through the entire hierarchy of items. These repeated exposures are generally done outside the therapy session, as homework done by the patients between sessions. This is then discussed and guided during the encounters with the therapists. Patients normally become more and more independent and autonomous, understanding through their own experiences what works for them in the exposure therapy and how they can use these strategies in other feared situations. Practice of in vivo exposure outside the therapeutic sessions is a key element for the success of the therapy. Habitually at least two to three exposure sessions are programmed with the patients: but the more frequent the exercises are, the more effective and rapid is the therapy. Situational exposures vary in accordance with the anxiety-provoking cues and the diagnostic of the patients. Table 5 describes some of classical exposure exercises for various anxious states.

Table 5. Examples of exposure exercises for various types of anxiety disorders

Anxiety disorder	Exposure exercises
Panic	Running up and down stairs. Turning on a chair to the point of dizziness.
Agoraphobia	Taking the bus from one station to the next. Walking through a supermarket and buying something.
Social phobia	Speaking in a group of persons. Asking for information at a desk.
Obsessive compulsive disorder	Leaving the apartment without verifying if all the lights are switched off. Touching a piece of dirty laundry without washing one's hands.
Post-traumatic stress disorder	Exposure to the memories of the traumatic event (emotional reliving of an accident, a funeral, scenes of violence during childhood). Exposure to objects and situations that are avoided, even if they do not represent any current danger.
Generalized anxiety disorder	Thinking of a problem that happens during a trip (automobile break down). Thinking of losing one's job.

4.2. Cognitive Interventions

Cognitive interventions can also take multiple forms and be based on various intervention techniques. Beck's approach, most likely the best known, organizes the therapeutic work around automatic thoughts, schemas and cognitive distortions (Beck and Emery, 1985; Beck et al., 1979). Using the Socratic dialogue (Taylor, 2000), the therapist identifies the automatic thoughts and progressively interrogates their logical distortions, before he brings to light the underlying beliefs and discusses their probable origin and their rationality or utility for the current circumstances. The key message upheld by the therapist is that the catastrophic interpretations of a situation (more than the situation itself) render it unpleasant and worsen the anxiety (Clark, 1986). It is possible through careful discussion about them and through corrective exercises to change the way the patient thinks about his feared situations and consequently to modify his feelings towards and during them. The basic idea of cognitive interventions is to challenge the distorted thoughts and beliefs through discussion or various forms of exercises / experiences, in order to replace them with more realistic and adaptive ones that can relieve from anxiety and give sufficient self-confidence.

Cognitive restructuring follows three to four major steps. Firstly the patient is informed about the assumptions of cognitive therapy through simple examples taken from ordinary life and from his own experiences. Once he is convinced of the link between thoughts and emotions, particularly in the sense that thoughts can influence emotions, the second step consists in identifying the automatic thoughts related to the feared situations. The patient evokes here all the catastrophic interpretations running through his head when he feels anxious or panicky. The therapist tries to discover what the antecedent stimuli are and especially what dangers do they represent for his client. This allows to understand the reasons for fear in the client's mind.

These interpretations are then questioned with the aim to stress the cognitive distortions they manifest. Through logical reasoning, therapist and client should conclude that the thoughts are in fact misinterpretations of the situation, and that they must be corrected, because they induce a lot of suffering and because alternative explanations also exist. The patient learns here to relativize the pertinence of his thoughts. He's invited to systematically ask himself if his anxious thoughts reflect reality or can they be challenged by alternative interpretations that could also correspond to the situation. It is absolutely necessary that the patient is intimately convinced of the logical errors present in his thoughts. He should agree for example with the idea that he exaggerates certain points and minimizes others, that he draws conclusions without veritable proof, or that he filters certain details of a situation to uphold his affirmations while forgetting other elements that could prove the contrary or support a different interpretation. This act of looking for alternative thoughts that are simultaneously more realistic and reassuring has a therapeutic impact by reducing tension and anxiety. But it also favours a sort of metacognitive process, where the patient progressively learns to criticize himself when he observes himself having dysfunctional attitudes. The individual becomes little by little able to identify his dysfunctional thoughts that provoke anxiety. He interiorly discusses them (or puts them on paper), and replaces them with anxiolytic thoughts. Different cognitive procedures exist, more or less standardized and more or less original and creative for realizing this work (McMullin, 2000). As the cognitive intervention progresses, the basic beliefs and the cognitive schemas are identified and discussed. At this point some authors make a distinction between maladaptive assumptions and dysfunctional schemas (Leahy and Holland, 2000). Assumptions are at a deeper level than automatic thoughts but not at the same fundamental level such as the schemas are. Assumptions are often expressed with "if... then..." or "I should..., to..." statements. Schemas or beliefs, as we have already said, represent more basic ideas about oneself, the others and the world. Statements are often affirmative and simple; they do not give rules or guides as the assumptions do. Table 6 gives some examples of automatic thoughts, assumptions and schemas. Such a distinction is however not always easy to grasp by patients (and sometimes by the therapist too!). It is our opinion that this distinction is not of fundamental importance for the success of the therapy. It seems nevertheless clear that the work on beliefs is very useful to favour a more fundamental change (helping perhaps by relapse prevention and self-management) that the transitory learning of compensatory coping strategies cannot do. With the modification of basic dysfunctional schemas, the individual certainly reduces his psychological vulnerability to anxiety and regains the necessary self-confidence to manage better stressful events and to maintain control over his physiological and emotional responses. Numerous books display lists of distorted thoughts, categories of logical distortions, and frequent or typical dysfunctional beliefs (Andrews et al., 2002; Babior and Goldman, 1997; Kozak and Foa, 1997; Leahy and Holland, 2000; White, 1999). Such books propose various targeted cognitive exercises too, which help the reader to modify his cognitive habits. They can be used as self-management guides for therapy or as a bibliotherapy tool completing the work done in sessions with a psychotherapist.

Table 6. Automatic thoughts, maladaptive assumptions and dysfunctional schemas by various types of anxiety disorders

Fear stimulus (activating event)	Automatic thought	Maladaptive assumption	Dysfunctional schemas
Panic she feels a slight sensation of dizziness while she is standing in line at a supermarket checkout	Here we go again! I need to go out immediately or I'll go insane.	If I don't control my anxiety, I will become psychotic and finish my life at the asylum.	The frontier between normality and madness is really tenuous.
Agoraphobia she's coming in the store	People see that I don't feel good.	I should never be weak, especially in normal situations such as going out to do some shopping.	People make fun of the ones that are weak.
Social phobia a man remains indifferent to her	He doesn't like me.	If I'm not an attractive woman for the men around me, I will remain alone.	I'm an unlovable woman.
Obsessive-compulsive disorder in front of a door of the medical office	Someone ill could have touched this door.	I should protect myself perfectly from any germ, especially AIDS, or I will die.	The world is full of invisible dangers. I could be very easily be contaminated by AIDS viruses.
Post-traumatic stress disorder image of one's dead son in a car accident	I'm guilty; I should be dead instead of my son.	I cannot be happy again without my son.	A guilty man must pay for his errors.
Generalized anxiety disorder before a dinner she's organizing	Everything will go wrong.	If I'm not completely prepared, I will fail.	I'm incompetent.

Other cognitive approaches appear more directive than cognitive restructuring. They propose one or another type of cognitive anxiety management methods to the client, by inviting him to take control again of his attentional and cognitive processes. These methods are essentially based on self-instructions, mental training and problem-solving skills. They are often elaborated and exercised in the office with the client before they are used in reality, during exposure exercises or during problematic situations. Table 7 summarizes such mental instructions, derived from the stress inoculation training method (Meichenbaum, 1977; Meichenbaum and Turk, 1976) that aims to improve the way one copes with one's anxiety.

Table 7. Self-Instructions Used To Cope With Anxiety-Inducing Situations

1. Preparation
What do I have to do?
I can prepare a plan of action.
I can succeed.
No negative comments! Think in a rational manner!
It is useless to worry too much. Worry will not improve anything; on the contrary it will worsen my present state.
Remember that avoiding fear only worsens it!
Don't do more or less than you've planned to do: it has to be a little difficult but not too much. It can't be too easy either; otherwise I won't make any progress.
I know I can do it, even if maybe it won't be perfect: what counts is that I do it.
2. Confrontation (exposure)
One step at a time, I'm putting myself to the test.
Try to not think too much about fear. It's better to concentrate on what you have to do.
Stay in contact with reality, don't close up on yourself.
What do you see around you? Is it really dangerous for you?
I can manage the situation; I am able, even if I feel intense fear.
3. Management of negative feelings
I can take a break if I feel too scared. But I mustn't leave the situation.
Remember what the therapist said: fear is nothing other than an emotion like any other, maybe more unpleasant, but certainly not unbearable or mortal. This is not the worst thing that can happen to me.
If I stay long enough in this situation, anxiety will go down. I will have won my bet and succeeded at my challenge.
If I evaluate my fear on a scale from 0 to 10. Where am I at now? Has it gone up or gone down? Why? Anyway, once 10 is reached my fear can't go any higher.
4. Reinforcements
Ok, well done. You did well. You're a champion!
It wasn't as bad as I thought it was going to be. I can do positive things even if I'm scared.
Was it really worth it to make such a fuss for this fear?
This experience will help me a lot for the future. Now I've understood that fear decreases with time as long as I stay in the situation.
The more I repeat this type of exercise, the better things will get.

Stress inoculation training takes place in three phases (Meichenbaum, 1996). 1) In the first phase (conceptualization phase) pedagogical work is done with the patient, during which he broadens his knowledge about fear and elaborates his own model in accounting for the specificity of his personal anxious problems. During the exchanges with his therapist, the patient is gently encouraged to view his fears and their triggering events as problems to be solved and not as unchangeable fatalistic events. 2) In the training phase the patient learns various methods of anxiety management: relaxation or breathing techniques, self-instructions, emotional self-soothing techniques, problem solving, interpersonal communication skills, etc.

He also learns to use these different methods by applying them mentally (for example by imagining that he is going through the stressful situation) or even by facing minor problems that are treatable in the therapist's office. The in-vivo training is gently introduced and tailored to the current competencies. 3) In the last phase (application phase), various opportunities to apply the new skills in real situations are searched for, according to a program which takes into account a gradually increasing level of skills needed to manage the situation. Personal experiments are carefully designed and prepared in order to be successfully coped with by the patient. Rehearsal, generalization procedures and relapse prevention interventions are also included in this phase. Stress inoculation training aims at providing the patient with an accessible and mastered repertoire of cognitive and behavioral skills that help him to cope with either various types of stressors or a particular specific difficulty.

4.3. Interventions at Physical Level

Methods of intervention acting on a physical and physiological level complete behavioral and cognitive methods. These methods are employed essentially for counteracting the physiological responses of anxiety. They provide the patients with simple and portable coping strategies to rapidly reduce or control tension and other physical symptoms. Diverse relaxation techniques can be applied. Passive methods, for example Schultz' autogenic training (Luthe and Schultz, 1969), often necessitate a quiet place, lying down or being seated; and generally require an auditory support that is verbal or musical. The individual is placed in a comfortable position and attentively listens to the therapist's instructions, with a soft agreeable music in the background. Progressively he will attain a state of tranquillity and relaxation, by simply following the given suggestions (for example "your arms become heavy and warm", "your body attains a state of relaxation", "the wrinkles on your forehead disappear", etc.). It is not even a rare event that the subject falls asleep when practising relaxation: in this case, the objective of total relaxation is perhaps certainly reached but it is then difficult to work with the person!

Active relaxation methods are at less risk of putting clients to sleep and are less demanding concerning the context: they can be practised virtually anywhere and at any time. In these methods, of which Jacobson's progressive method (1938) is a famous prototype, the individual learns to feel sensations of relaxation by differentiating them from feelings of tension (Barlow and Cerny, 1988; Leahy and Holland, 2000; Öst, 1987). The following sequence is habitually applied to various muscular groups: 1) during a few seconds the patient contracts as hard as possible the concerned group of muscles (for example: the hand, the forearm, the shoulders, etc.), 2) he releases the contracted muscles so that they loosen up progressively; during this phase he focuses his attention during 10 to 20 seconds on the physical sensations that emerge. Afterwards he can take a pause with a deep sigh, before repeating the sequence on the same or on another group of muscles. Specific movements are proposed in order to allow the individual to correctly contract the muscular group that he's working on: for example squeezing one's fist, shrugging one's shoulders, pushing one's tongue against the palate, etc. Once the patient has understood the different exercises and correctly recognizes the sensation of relaxation, he can simply associate these sensations to a word (for example "relax", "calm", etc.). This last phase is called the cue controlled relaxation, because the releasing of the muscles is associated with a particular cue (in this case a word). Through conditioning, these words will be able by themselves to set off calming reactions that were previously attained through the tension-relaxation exercises. Leahy and Holland (2000) propose for example a six-steps relaxation technique that brings the patients from a global relaxation to more focused relaxation and finally to a cue controlled relaxation (table 8).

Table 8. Six-Steps Relaxation Procedure For Coping With Anxiety And Tension (Leahy And Holland, 2000)

Step	Exercise
Twelve-muscle-group-relaxation	Application of the tense-relax technique to 12 groups of muscles: 1) lower arms, b) upper arms, 3) lower legs, 4) thighs, 5) stomach, 6) upper chest and back, 7) shoulders, 8) back of the necks, 9) lips, 10) eyes, 11) eyebrows, 12) upper forehead and scalp. The tense-relax technique follow this sequence: a) let the patient focus on breathing during two or three breaths; b) let tense a group of muscles during 5 seconds (counting from 1 to 5 is possible; it helps patients and therapists to give the rhythm of the exercise); c) let release the muscles and focus during 15-20 seconds on the sensations in these muscles (with helping instructions); d) repeat the procedure a-c for all groups of muscles; e) count down from 5 to 1 and give for every number a new relaxation suggestion; f) focus on breathing during 1 minute; g) count up from 1 to 5 while inviting the client to become alert again; h) let practice at home 2 times a day during 1-2 weeks (with and without audiotaped instructions).
Eight-muscle-group-relaxation	Same tense-relax procedure but limited to the eight following groups of muscles:1) whole arms, 2) whole legs, 3) stomach, 4) upper chest and back, 5) shoulders, 6) back of the neck, 7) face, 8) forehead and scalp. Time of the releasing period should be increased to at least 30 seconds.
Four-muscle-group-relaxation	Same tense-relax procedure but limited to only four groups of muscles: 1) whole arms, 2) upper chest and back, 3) shoulders and neck, 4) face. Vary the positions and the settings for the practice (waiting for the bus, during a pause at the office, walking, etc.).
Release-only relaxation	Relaxation of the same four-muscle-group as in the precedent step, but without the phase of tension: a) let the patient focus on one group of muscles (with noticing any tension), b) let the patient recall the sensation of relaxation and then release the tension (during 30-45 seconds), c) if the tension is totally absent, proceed to the next group of muscles, d) when the person is fully relaxed, proceed as usual with the counting down and counting up procedure.
Cue controlled relaxation	1. Application of the release-only relaxation When relaxed let the patient take deep breaths and say "relax" at each exhalation while releasing any tension that could be detected. 2. Application of the breathing and saying "relax" phase without the release-only procedure. 3. Application of the cue controlled relaxation 10-15 times each day
Practice in stressful situations	Apply the relaxation technique in more and more stressful situations, especially when first signs of anxiety appear.

Relaxation methods are very useful and often highly appreciated. They frequently improve the sensation of well-being. Nevertheless they require rigorous training during 2 to 4 weeks, before being able to self-control them and to benefit fully from their effects. Some patients are incapable, especially in a state of anxiety or in crisis situations, of learning or practising them. It is not rare to observe that relaxation techniques even have a paradoxical effect by inducing anxiety in patients who practise it (Heide and Borkevec, 1984). This is why briefer methods, that are simpler forms of relaxation, have been proposed as a physical adjuvant to the management of anxiety. We can mention here in particular different breathing methods and vaso-vagal techniques that permit to lower heart-rate (Bannister, 1983; Satory and Olajide, 1988). The individual can in this way control the frequency and amplitude of his breathing: he can thusly learn to regulate its frequency (by counting for example from 1 to 3 at each inspiration and each expiration), to block it a few seconds after inspiration, or to find an agreeable rhythm (Leahy and Holland, 2000). It is important here to make a clear understandable difference between "chest breathing" and "diaphragm breathing" and to help the patient to learn a diaphragmatic breathing (Taylor, 2000).

5. Effectiveness of Cognitive-Behavioral Treatements: A Brief Overview

Cognitive behavior therapies have achieved very good results in controlled outcome studies. Numerous literature reviews and meta-analyses have synthesized a large amount of studies. Specific phobias were historically the first disorders that behavioral therapies treated. The results have always been positive and encouraging: exposure to phobic stimuli (with the corresponding processes of habituation and extinction) has been widely demonstrated as an effective way to reduce such phobias (Andrews et al., 2002). A debate has been devoted to the question of the usefulness of cognitive elements in therapy. Do they improve the results of the behavioral interventions? No definitive answer can be made, because some empirical results have contradicted this view, while the theoretical model and some other studies have tended to support it (Andrews, 2002; Beck et al., 1985).

For panic and agoraphobia the meta-analytic reviews conclude that cognitive behavior therapies are well tolerated, moderately to highly effective, and certainly represent the most effective treatment amongst psychological interventions (Taylor, 2000). However other psychotherapies seem to have been insufficiently studied to seriously conclude to the superiority of cognitive behavior therapy for panic disorder and agoraphobia. But in the current situation of incomplete knowledge about the effectiveness of other forms of psychotherapy, cognitive behavioral treatment appears as the treatment of choice for these syndromes. This is particularly true for new treatment packages specifically designed for panic disorder and agoraphobia (often called the second generation of cognitive behavior therapy or CBT2). Such therapeutic programs focus their interventions on the panic processes, by correcting the cognitive catastrophic misinterpretations of internal stimuli and by offering exposure to body sensations rather than exposure to external fear stimuli (Barlow and Cerny, 1988; Clark and Salkovskis, 1987; Craske, Meadows and Barlow, 1994). Chambless and Gillis (1993, 1994) find in their meta-analytic study that such treatment packages have lower attrition rates (8%) than applied relaxation alone (12%) or in-vivo exposure alone (16%). Moreover, 88% patients having had CBT2 were free of panic at the end of treatment (61% for applied relaxation group, 54% for the exposure group and 12% for the waiting list group). In comparison with pharmacological treatments, CBT2 interventions do not clearly appear superior at posttreatement, but their strength lies in the long-term effects. In fact long-term follow-up studies (from 2 to 6 years) show that exposure treatments and cognitive-behavior therapies of the second generation maintain their gains through the time and are thus likely to be more effective than short-term pharmacotherapies (Taylor, 2000). These results are easy to interpret: psychological treatment favours cognitive and emotional restructuring and give coping strategies and management techniques that medication cannot offer! If drug treatment is conducted without these psychological adjuvants, nothing is learned by the patient, and the emotional problems are more likely to reappear once the pharmacological intervention is stopped.

For social phobics, cognitive behavior therapies have proved also to be superior to placebo treatments or waiting lists. Combined treatments including cognitive interventions and subject's exposure to social situations with social skills training seem to be more effective than treatment offering only isolated components (Taylor, 1996), especially if the outcome at follow-up (3 to 6 months) is taken into consideration. Few studies have assessed the impact of cognitive behavior therapy on a long-term basis. Heimberg and colleagues reported at 4.5 to 6.5 years after treatment, superior results for cognitive behavior interventions in comparison with a therapeutic package composed by education and supportive psychotherapy (Heimberg, Dodge, Hope, Kennedy, and Zollo, 1990; Heimberg, Salzman, Holt, and Blendell, 1993). The group format can be preferred to individual therapy: the group itself realizes an intrinsic exposure to social contacts. Such an exposure is not always easy to create, because of the often unexpected or brief nature of social situations and interpersonal interactions (Butler, 1989): the group situation therefore appears as a good opportunity to do it. However there is no definitive scientific evidence that the group format results in better outcomes than the individual format (Gould, Buckminster, Pollack, Otto, and Yap, 1997). Needless to say that the economic and intrinsic advantages of the group format habitually make the therapists prefer it.

There is again wide agreement that cognitive behavior therapies provide substantial relief and clinically and statistically significant improvement for patients suffering from generalized anxiety disorders (Borkovec and Whisman, 1996; Fisher and Durham, 1999; Gould, Otto, Pollack, and Yap, 1997). This active approach is clearly superior to non treatment conditions and to nondirective therapies (Durham, Fisher, Treliving, Hau, Richard, and Stewart, 1999; Durham, Murphy, Allan, Richard, Treliving, and Fenton, 1994). Cognitive interventions aim for better tolerance of uncertainty and the correction of erroneous beliefs about worry or cognitive avoidance while behavioral techniques use in particular relaxation methods and problem solving skills training. Both methods have proved to be effective (Borkovec and Costello, 1993; Ladouceur, Dugas, Freeston, Léger, Gagnon, and Thibodeau, 2000; Öst and Breitholtz, 2000). As with specific phobias or social phobias, the debate about the question of the active components of the therapy, here expressed in the comparison between relaxation procedures and cognitive behavioral oriented programs, remains open. If for theoretical reasons cognitive behavior therapies seem to be preferred to purely behavioral interventions, empirical evidence doesn't support such an affirmation (Andrews et al., 2002). Data are nevertheless lacking that could allow to pose a clear differential indication for every sort of treatment.

Various treatment options can be offered to patients suffering from post-traumatic stress disorder. These options combine cognitive and behavioral components in various ways, stressing on anxiety management techniques, exposure to traumatic memories or cognitive restructuring. Anxiety management techniques are mostly derived from the Stress Inoculation Training (Meichenbaum, 1985): they try to provide the patients with coping strategies for the physical (relaxation and breathing training), behavioral (various skills training to improve assertiveness and to help patients to resume the disrupted daily activities) and cognitive domains (such as thought stopping or distraction techniques to gain control over unexpected and distressing memories). Prolonged exposure treatments have been demonstrated in controlled trials as marginally superior to anxiety management programs, especially at follow-up measures (12 months), with around 60% of improvement in severity of the disorder for (Foa, Dancu, Hembree, Jaycox, Meadows, and Street, 1999, Foa, Rothbaum, Riggs, and Murdock, 1991). Resick and Schnicke (1993) have proposed and evaluated a more cognitive oriented therapy, called Cognitive Processing Therapy: cognitive restructuring techniques focus on five primary themes in post-traumatic stress problems: safety, trust, power, self-esteem and intimacy. Results are encouraging (with 40-55% improvement at post-treatment), but perhaps not as effective as exposure treatments, where very good results have been more recently found with improvement rates varying between 65 to 80% (Resick, and Schnicke, 1992; Richards, Lovell and Marks, 1994; Thompson, Charlton, Kerry, and Lee, 1995). Controlled studies have then provided favourable results for the cognitive behavioral treatment of post-traumatic stress disorder. However it appears relatively difficult to differentiate between programs, because studies did not always have targeted the same population (i.e. suffering from similar traumatic events). As a rule of thumb, Andrews et al. (2002) propose that cognitive behavior therapy for post-traumatic stress disorder improves around two thirds of the patients, with 30% doing very well after a follow-up period of one year.

Behavioral therapies based on the prolonged exposure to obsessional cues with response prevention of the rituals have been largely documented and considered as the recommended treatment for obsessive compulsive disorders. One can expect at posttreatment until 60% to 70% of improvement in the severity of rituals by half the patients who complete the treatment (Foa, Steketee, and Ozarow, 1985). We can expect improvements to be maintained at 3 years, with an approximate dropout rate of 10%: in a follow-up study 78% of the patients who completed the treatment remained improved after a period of 3 years, with an average of 60% of improvement in the targeted rituals (O'Sullivan, Noshirvani, Marks, Montiero, and Lelliot, 1991). However we have to keep in mind that around a quarter of patients may refuse treatment, because of time commitment and fear of being confronted to obsessions without being able to cope with anxiety (Greist, 1998). Motivational adjunctions and carefully elaborated hierarchies of cues can overcome the problem of accepting the treatment, but they increase the treatment duration. Cognitive procedures have also been under empirical investigation. Van Oppen and colleagues found for example that cognitive therapy and self-controlled exposure led to similar results: significant improvements were observed in both groups, with perhaps a tendency to do better by the cognitive intervention group (van Oppen, de Haan, van Balkom, Spinhoven, Hoogduin, and van Dyck, 1995). Finally psychosocial therapies including cognitive-behavioral interventions and pharmacotherapy are also considered by clinicians as a good treatment strategy, because of probable synergetic effects of medication and psychological interventions for the symptom reduction and the relapse prevention. However there aren't any definitive results about a possible additive effect: current studies indicate that both strategies are equally effective but that the combination of the two does not significantly improve the results of the therapies alone (Kobak, Greist,

Jeffersen, Katzelnick, and Henk, 1998). Therefore the choice of a treatment remains clearly in the hands of the therapists (and theirs clients) who have access to cognitive, behavioral and pharmacological interventions in order to administer the different therapies they propose to their patients.

6. Conclusion

Fear is a central feature in human emotional life and this emotional state is perfectly normal. The psychophysiological process of anxiety tends naturally to maintain this emotion through avoidance mechanisms that reinforce it. The mechanisms of fear are particularly efficient in the case of real danger, because they help the organism to be rapidly prepared and immediately react in front of a real danger. Fear becomes pathological when it appears in non dangerous situations, when it is maintained by these normal psycho-biological mechanisms, impeding the person the overcome his emotions, and creating suffering and handicaps that can be invasive and insuperable.

The cognitive-behavioral models of fear and anxiety disorders are based on the classical syndromes described by international classifications of psychiatric disorders, such as the DSM-IV or the ICD-10. Using learning paradigms (associative learning and operant conditioning) they stress the role of the environmental and the behavioral components of the fear process: they show how association between fear and situations can transform neutral stimuli in anxiety-provoking stimuli; they also show how escape and avoidance behaviors reinforce the anxiety response. The cognitive part of these models stresses the role of efficacy and outcome expectancies in the behavioural choices, the impact of the attentional processes in the anxiety response, and the link between automatic distorted thoughts, their underlying beliefs and the emotions they can trigger.

These theoretical models, issued essentially from experimental psychology, social psychology and neuropsychology, have provided new insights of the phenomenon and have brought new ideas for treatment methods. Today, therapists have a relatively vast arsenal of intervention methods. Techniques of cognitive behavior therapy can be classified in three broad categories: 1) behavioral interventions which essentially include exposure with response prevention techniques, 2) cognitive interventions which can be subdivided in cognitive restructuring (working on automatic thoughts and underlying beliefs), self-instructional training (to modify coping strategies and attentional processes), and working on self-efficacy expectancies, 3) physical interventions such as breathing retraining or relaxation methods. Currently, treatments for anxiety rarely use in fact one type of intervention at a time. They rather combine diverse ingredients. It is up to the therapist to adjust as well as possible these diverse interventions to the characteristics of the patient and to formulate a pertinent and efficient sequence therapeutic strategy.

Therapeutic plans usually align themselves with the following structure (according to Andrews et al., 2002; Barlow and Cerny, 1988; Leahy and Holland, 2000): 1) investigation and assessment (including diagnostic, functional analysis of fear □gimuli, behaviors, affect, cognitions, and consequences), 2) information about the disorder and its treatment, 3) proposal of treatment, 4) application of treatment (where its components are defined in phase 3), 5) evaluation of the efficiency of the interventions, 6) end of treatment (with work on relapse prevention, eventual "booster" sessions, and final evaluation). From now on the models of the general conception of anxiety and the intervention methods can be adapted to each specific anxiety disorder, with the goal of ameliorating their pertinence and efficiency.

Numerous manuals and self-help books have been edited to aid therapists and patients to structure their therapy (Andrews et al., 2002; Babior and Goldman, 1997; Barlow and Cerny, 1988; Kozak and Foa, 1997; Leahy and Holland, 2000; White, 1999). They generally present the current models of anxiety in a didactical way, often with simple words so that anyone can understand the theoretical background of the therapy. With this in mind, they display tables with lists of symptoms, avoidance behaviours, distorted thoughts, their related categories of logical distortions, and classical dysfunctional beliefs. Therapeutic interventions are described step by step, and various charts, diagrams and working sheets complete these descriptions and give to the reader all that is necessary to begin self-therapy.

In more classical psychotherapy, the therapist guides his patient during the treatment process. He helps to diagnose the anxiety disorder; he elaborates with his client the therapeutic hypothesis and proposes what could be the treatment of choice for him. In behavioral and physical interventions the therapist adopts the role of a coach training his client in correctly making the exposure and in adequately learning the relaxation method. In cognitive interventions, he appears more as a gentle conversation companion, bringing to light the relationships between thoughts and emotions, and questioning the relevance of some automatic thoughts and beliefs. He never imposes his modes of thinking; he rather helps his client to discover new beliefs that appear more appropriate to him. He functions like a philosophical guide, searching more, like Socrates, to reflect upon thought processes that intervene in the anxiety problem, instead of giving recipes for positively thinking. This humble attitude of collaboration that characterizes the cognitive-behavior therapist isn't the only attitude he adopts. In fact, in order to correctly achieve his work he must equally present–beyond his qualities of listening, collaboration, warmth, empathy and flexibility–a professional attitude. He has to show his mastering of the theoretical knowledge and techniques in the pathologies he treats, and his capacity to structure a treatment in a coherent way, for an individual session as well as for the length of an entire treatment (Blackburn and Davidson, 1980).

If most of the anxiety disorders can be treated with cognitive behavior therapies with reasonable positive expectancies regarding the outcome, some limitations have to be mentioned here. First of all, we need more long-term outcome studies that prove permanent achievement of the gains years after the treatment. The aim of the cognitive behavior therapy is to develop self-management skills by the patients, so that they can use in the future what they have learned in therapy to prevent the relapse or the recurrence of the disorders. If relapse is impossible to avoid, previous therapies should lead the patients to need less therapy and professional help in this occasion. Such results still have to be demonstrated. Secondly, we need to better our knowledge of what the really the active components of treatment are. Today the comparisons between cognitive and behavioral interventions have not allowed clinicians to reach any definitive conclusion in this debate; often isolated elements are equally effective, and the combination of therapies does not always prove to be better than the interventions alone. Thirdly, we also need more results about the outcome of other forms of therapy for anxiety disorders. Only pharmacological and cognitive behavioral treatments have been scientifically studied. That's also the reason why they are the treatments of choice today in modern psychiatry. Nevertheless a panacea does not exist for the treatment of anxiety disorders. Cognitive behavior therapies are surely the current treatments of choice, but progress can still be made to improve not only the clinical outcomes for patients, but also the theoretical knowledge about this central emotion in the life of human beings.

BIBLIOGRAPHY

American Psychiatric Association. (1994). *Diagnostic and Statistical Manual of Mental Disorders (4th edition)*. Washington DC: Author.

Andrews, G., Creamer, M., Crino, R., Hunt, C., Lampe, L., and Page, A. (2002). *The treatment of anxiety disorders. Clinician guides and patient manuals*. Cambridge: Cambridge University Press.

Babior, S., and Goldman, C. (1997). *A 10-week recovery program for overcoming panic, anxiety and phobias*. La Jolla, CA: Whole Person Press.

Bandura, A. (1977). *Social learning theory*. New York: Prentice-Hall.

Bandura, A. (1986). *Social foundations of thought and action. A social cognitive theory*. Englewood Cliffs, NJ: Prentice-Hall.

Bandura, A. (1988). Self-efficacy conception of anxiety. *Anxiety research, 1*(2), 77-98.

Bannister, R. (1983). *Autonomic failure*. Oxford: Oxford University Press.

Barlow, D. H. (1988). *Anxiety and its disorders. The nature and treatment of anxiety and panic*. New York, NY: The Guilford Press.

Barlow, D. H., and Cerny, J. A. (1988). *Psychological treatment of panic*. New York, NY: The Guilford Press.

Beck, A. T., and Emery, G. (1985). *Anxiety disorders and phobias: a cognitive perspective*. New York: Basic Books.

Beck, A. T., Rush, J., Shaw, B., and Emery, G. (1979). *Cognitive therapy of depression*. New York: Guilford Press.

Bijl, R. V., Ravelli, A., and van Zessen, G. (1998). Prevalence of psychiatric disorder in the general population: results of The Netherlands Mental Health Survey and Incidence Study (NEMESIS). *Social Psychiatry and Psychiatric Epidemiology, 33*(12), 587-595.

Blackburn, I.-M. (1992). *Coping with depression* (reprinted ed.). Edinburgh: Chambers.

Blackburn, I.-M., and Davidson, K. (1990). *Cognitive therapy for depression and anxiety*. Oxford: Blackwell Scientific Publications.

Borkovec, T. D., and Whisman, M. A. (1996). Psychosocial treatment for generalized anxiety disorder. In M. R. Mavissakalian and R. F. Prien (Eds.), *Long-term treatments of anxiety disorders* (pp. 171-199). Washington, DC: American Psychiatric Press.

Brown, T. A., DiNardo, P., and Barlow, D. H. (1994). *ADIS - Anxiety Disorders Interview Schedule for DSM IV. Adult and Lifetime combination kit*. Boulder, CO: Graywind Publications Incorporated.

Brown, T. A., Marten, P. A., and Barlow, D. H. (1995). Discriminant validity of the symptoms constituting the DSM-III-R an DSM-IV associated symptoms criterion of generalized anxiety disorder. *Journal of Anxiety Disorders, 9*, 317-328.

Butler, G. (1989). Issues in the application of cognitive and behavioral strategies in the treatement of social phobia. *Clinical Psychology Review, 9*, 91-106.

Chambless, D. L., and Gillis, M. M. (1993). Cognitive therapy of anxiety disorders. *Journal of Consulting and Clinical Psychology, 61*, 248-260.

Chambless, D. L., and Gillis, M. M. (1994). A review of psychosocial treatments for panic disorder. In B. E. Wolfe and M. J. D. (Eds.), *Treatment of panic disorder: a consensus development conference* (pp. 149-173). Washington, DC: American Psychiatric Press.

Clark, D. M. (1986). A cognitive approach to panic. *Behavior Research and Therapy, 24*(4), 461-470.

Clark, D. A., and Salkovskis, P. M. (1987). *Cognitive therapy for panic attacks: therapist's manual*. Oxford: Departement of Psychiatry, University of Oxford.

Clark, D.M., and Wells, A. (1995) A cognitive model of social phobia. In R.G. Heimberg, M. Liebowitz, D. Hope, and F. Scheier (Eds) *Social Phobia: Diagnosis, Assessment, and Treatment* (pp 69-93). New York: The Guilford Press.

Connor-Smith, J. K., and Compas, B. E. (2002). Vulnerability to social stress: Coping as a mediator or moderator of sociotropy and symptoms of anxiety and depression. *Cognitive Therapy and Research, 26*(1), 39-55.

Craske, M. G., Meadows, E. A., and Barlow, D. H. (1994). *Mastery of you anxiety and panic II and agoraphobia supplement: therapist guide*. San Antonio, TX: Psychological Corporation.

Durham, R. C., Fisher, P. L., Treliving, L. R., Hau, C. M., Richard, K., and Stewart, J. B. (1999). One year follow-up of cognitive therapy, analytic psychotherapy and anxiety management training for generalized anxiety disorder: Symptom change, medication usage and attitudes to treatment. *Behavioural and Cognitive Psychotherapy, 27*(1), 19-35.

Durham, R. C., Murphy, T., Allan, T., Richard, K., Treliving, L. R., and Fenton, G. W. (1994). Cognitive therapy, analytic psychotherapy and anxiety management training for generalised anxiety disorder. *British Journal of Psychiatry, 36*, 101-119.

Ekman, P. (1994). *The nature of emotion: fundamental questions*. New York: Oxford University Press.

Emmelkamp, P. M. E., and Wessels, D. H. (1975). Flooding in imgination vs flooding in vivo: a comparision with agoraphobics. *Behavior Research and Therapy, 13*, 7-15.

Fiegenbaum, W. (1988). Long-term efficacy of ungraded versus graded massed exposure in agoraphobics. In I. Hand and H. U. Wittchen (Eds.), *Panic and phobias. Treatments and variables affecting course and outcome* (pp. 83-88). Berlin: Springer-Verlag.

Fisher, P. L., and Durham, R. C. (1999). Recovery rates in generalized anxiety disorders following psychological therapy: an analysis of clinically significant change in the STAI-T across outcome studies since 1990. *Psychological Medicine, 29*, 1425-1434.

Foa, E. B., Dancu, C. V., Hembree, E. A., Jaycox, L. H., Meadows, E. A., and Street, G. P. (1999). A comparison of exposure therapy, stress inoculation training, and their combination for reducing posttraumatic stress disorder in female assault victims. *Journal of Consulting and Clinical Psychology, 67*(2), 194-200.

Foa, E., and Kozak, M. J. (1986). Emotional processing of fear: exposure to corrective information. *Psychological Bulletin, 99*, 20-35.

Foa, E. B., Rothbaum, B. O., Riggs, D. S., and Murdock, T. B. (1991). Treatment of posttraumatic stress disorder in rape victims: a comparison between cognitive-behavioral procedures and counseling. *Journal of Consulting and Clinical Psychology, 59*(5), 715-723.

Foa, E. B., Steketee, G. S., and Ozarow, B. J. (1985). Behaviour therapy with obsessive-compulsives: from therapy to treatment. In M. Mavissakalian and S. M. Turner and M. Michelsen (Eds.), *Obsessive-compulsive disorder: psychological and pharmacological treatments*. New York: Plenum Press.

Friedman, E. S., Clark, D. B., and Gershon, S. (1992). Stress, anxiety, and depression: Review of biological, diagnostic, and nosologic issues. *Journal of Anxiety Disorders, 6*(4), 337-363.

Goldberg, D. P., and Lecrubier, Y. (1995). Form and frequency of mental disorders across centres. In T. B. Ustun and N. Sartorius (Eds.), *Mental illness in general health care: An international study* (pp. 323–334). New York: John Wiley and Sons.

Gould, R. A., Buckminster, S., Pollack, M. H., Otto, M. W., and Yap, L. (1997). Cognitive-behavioral and pharmacological treatment for social phobia: A meta-analysis. *Clinical Psychology Science and Practice, 4*(4), 291-306.

Gould, R. A., Otto, M. W., Pollack, M. H., and Yap, L. (1997). Cognitive behavioral and pharmacological treatment of generalized anxiety disorder: A preliminary meta-analyis. *Behavior Therapy, 28*(2), 285-305.

Grawe, K., Donati, R., and Bernauer, F. (1994). *Psychotherapie im Wandel. Von der Konfession zur Profession*. Bern: Hogrefe.

Gray, J. A. (1991). *The Psychology of fear and stress* (2th ed. reprinted with corrections ed.). Cambridge: Cambridge University Press.

Greist, J. H. (1998). The comparative effectiveness of treatments for obsessive-compulsive disorder. *Bulletin of the Menninger Clinic, 62*(suppl. A), A65-A81.

Heide, F. J., and Borkovec, T. D. (1984). Relaxation-induced anxiety: Mechanisms and theoretical implications. *Behavior Research and Therapy, 22*(1), 1-12.

Heimberg, R. G., Dodge, C. S., Hope, D. A., Kennedy, C. R., and Zollo, L. J. (1990). Cognitive behavioral group treatment for social phobia: Comparison with a credible placebo control. *Cognitive Therapy and Research, 14*(1), 1-23.

Heimberg, R. G., Salzman, D. G., Holt, C. S., and Blendell, K. A. (1993). Cognitive-behavioral group treatment for social phobia: Effectiveness at five-year followup. *Cognitive Therapy and Research, 17*(4), 325-339.

Himadi, W. G., and et al. (1986). The relationship of marital adjustment to agoraphobia treatment outcome. *Behavior Research and Therapy, 24*(2), 107-115.

Ingram, R. E., Miranda, J., and Segal, Z. V. (1998). *Cognitive vulnerability to depression.* New York: The Guilford Press.

Jacobson, E. (1974). *Progressive relaxation: A physiological and clinical investigation of muscular states and their significance in psychology and medical practice*. Chicago, IL: University of Chicago Press.

Jannoun, L., Munby, M., Catalan, J., and Gelder, M. (1980). A home-based treatment program for agoraphobia: Replication and controlled evaluation. *Behavior Therapy, 11*(3), 294-305.

Kanfer, F. H., and Saslow, G. (1969). Behavioral diagnosis. In C. M. Franks (Ed.), *Behavior therapy: appraisal and status* (pp. 417-444). New York: MacGraw Hill.

Kanfer, F. H., and Schefft, B. (1988). *Guiding the process of therapeutic change*. Champaign, IL: Research Press.

Kobak, K. A., Greist, J. H., Jeffersen, J. W., Katzelnick, D. J., and Henk, H. J. (1998). Behavioral versus pharmacological treatments of obsessive-compulsive disorder: a meta-analysis. *Psychopharmacology, 136*, 205-216.

Kopta, S. M., Lueger, R. J., Saunders, S. M., and Howard, K. I. (1999). Individual psychotherapy outcome and process research: challenges leading to greater turmoil or a positive transition? *Annual Review of Psychology., 50*, 441-469.

Kozak, M. J., and Foa, E. B. (1997). *Mastery of obsessive-compulsive disorder. A cognitive-behavioral approach*. Boulder, CO: Graywind Publications Incorporated.

Ladouceur, R., Dugas, M. J., Freeston, M. H., Leger, E., Gagnon, F., and Thibodeau, N. (2000). Efficacy of a cognitive-behavioral treatment for generalized anxiety disorder: evaluation in a controlled clinical trial. *Journal of Consulting and Clinical Psychology, 68*(6), 957-964.

Laitinen-Krispijn, S., and Bijl, R. V. (2000). Mental disorders and employee sickness absence: the NEMESIS study. Netherlands Mental Health Survey and Incidence Study. *Social Psychiatry and Psychiatric Epidemiology, 35*(2), 71-77.

Lang, P. J. (1984). Cognition in emotion: concept and action. In C. Izard and J. Kagan and R. Zajonc (Eds.), *Emotions, cognition, and behavior*. New York: Cambridge University Press.

Leahy, R. L., and Holland, S. J. (2000). *Treatment plans and interventions for depression and anxiety disorders*. New York: The Guilford Press.

Luthe, W., and Schultz, J. H. (1969). *The autogenic Therapy. Vol 1. Autogenic methods*. New York: Grune and Stratton Inc.

Mackintosh, N. J. (1983). *Conditioning and associative learning*. New York: Oxford University Press.

Magee, W. J., Eaton, W. W., Wittchen, H. U., McGonagle, K. A., and Kessler, R. C. (1996). Agoraphobia, simple phobia, and social phobia in the National Comorbidity Survey. *Archives of General Psychiatry, 53*(2), 159-168.

Marks, I. M. (1987). *Fears, phobias and rituals: panic, anxiety and their disorders*. New York: Oxford University Press.

Marsland, D. W., Wood, M., and Mayo, F. (1976). Content of family practice: a data bank for patient care, curriculum and research in family practice. *Journal of Family Practice, 3*, 25-68.

Marten, P. A., Brown, T. A., Barlow, D. H., Borkovec, T. D., Shear, M. K., and Lydiard, R. B. (1993). Evaluation of the ratings comprising the associated symptoms criterion DSM-III-R generalized anxiety disorder. *Journal of Nervous and Mental Disease, 181*, 676-682

Matthews, A. M., Johnston, D. W., Lancashire, M., Munby, M., Shaw, P. N., and Gelder, M. (1976). Imaginal flooding and exposure to real phobic situations: treatment outcome with agoraphobic patients. *British Journal of Psychiatry, 129*, 362-371.

McMullin, R. E. (2000). *The new handbook of cognitive therapy techniques*. New York: W.W. Norton and Company.

Meichenbaum, D. (1977). *Cognitive-behavior modification. An integrative approach*. New York: Plenum Press.

Meichenbaum, D. (1985). *Stress inoculation training*. New York: Pergamon Press.

Meichenbaum, D. (1996). Stress inoculation training for coping with stressors. *The Clinical Psychologist, 49*, 4-7.

Meichenbaum, D., and Turk, D. (1976). The cognitive-behavioral management of anxiety, anger and pain. In P. Davidson (Ed.), *The Behavioral Management of Anxiety, Depression and Pain*. New York: Brunner/Mazel.

Mowrer, O. H. (1960). *Learning theory and behavior*. New York: Wiley.

National Institute of Mental Health Molecular Genetics Initiative. (1992). *Diagnostic Interview For Genetic Studies (DIGS) - version 2.0*. Bethesda: National Institute of Mental Health.

Ortony, A., and Turner, T. J. (1990). What's basic about basic emotions? *Psychological Review, 97*(3), 315-331.

Öst, L.-G. (1987). Applied relaxation: Description of a coping technique and review of controlled studies. *Behavior Research and Therapy, 25*(5), 397-409.

Öst, L. G., and Breitholtz, E. (2000). Applied relaxation vs. cognitive therapy in the treatment of generalized anxiety disorder. *Behaviour Research and Therapy, 38*(8), 777-790.

O'Sullivan, G., Noshirvani, H., Marks, I. M., Montiero, W., and Lelliot, P. (1991). Six year follow-up after exposure and clomipramine therapy for obsessive compulsive disorder. *Journal of Clinical Psychiatry, 52*, 150-155.

Peter, H., and Hand, I. (1988). Patterns of patient-spouse interaction n agoraphobics: assessment by Camberwelle Family Interview (CFI) and impact on outcome of self-exposure treatment. In I. Hand and H.-U. Wittchen (Eds.), *Panic and phobias 2. Treatments and variables affecting course and outcome* (pp. 240-251). Berlin: Springer-Verlag.

Pollard, C. A., Henderson, J. G., Frank, M., and Margolis, R. B. (1989). Help-seeking patterns of anxiety-disordered individuals in the general population. *Journal of Anxiety Disorders, 3*(3), 131-138.

Rachman, S. (1978). *Fear and courage*. San Francisco: W.H. Freeman.

Rachman, S. (1980). Emotional processing. *Behavior Research and Therapy, 18*, 51-60.

Rachman, S. (1998). Panic and anxiety. In S. Rachman (Ed.), *Anxiety* (pp. 87-113). Hove: Psychology Press.

Rees, C. S., Richards, J. C., and Smith, L. M. (1998). Medical utilisation and costs in panic disorder: a comparison with social phobia. *Journal of Anxiety Disorders, 12*(5), 421-435.

Rescorla, R. A. (1988). Pavlovian conditioning. It's not what you think it is. *American Psychologist, 43*(3), 151-160.

Resick, P. A., and Schnicke, M. K. (1992). Cognitive processing therapy for sexual assault victims. *Journal of Consulting and Clinical Psychology, 60*(5), 748-756.

Resick, P. A., and Schnicke, M. K. (1993). *Cognitive Processing Therapy for sexual assault victims: a treatment manual*. Newbury Park, CA: Sage Publications.

Richards, D. A., Lovell, K., and Marks, I. M. (1994). Post-traumatic stress disorder: evaluation of a behavioral treatment program. *Journal of Traumatic Stress, 7*, 669-680.

Robins, L. N., Cottler, L. B., Buchholz, K. K., Compton, W. M., North, C. S., and Rourke, K. N. (2000). *Diagnostic Interview Schedule for the DSM-IV (DIS-IV)*. St. Louis, MO: Washington University School of Medicine.

Robinson, E. L., Corbett, M. O., and Spurlock, H. (1996). The effects of physical and mental stress on cardiovascular reactivity in a group of African American female college students. *Journal of Anxiety Disorders, 10*(6), 543-553.

Salkovskis, P. M. (Ed.). (1996). *The frontiers of cognitive therapy*. New York: Guilford Press.

Salkovskis, P. M., Clark, D. M., Hackmann, A., Wells, A., and Gelder, M. G. (1999). An experimental investigation of the role of safety-seeking behaviors in the maintenance of panic disorder with agoraphobia. *Behavior Research and Therapy, 37*(6), 559-574.

Sartory, G., and Olajide, D. (1988). Vagal innervation techniques in the treatment of panic disorder. *Behavior Research and Therapy, 26*(5), 431-434.

Scheier, M. F., Carver, C. S., and Matthews, K. A. (1983). Attentional factors in the perception of bodily states. In J. T. Cacioppo and R. E. Petty (Eds.), *Social psychophysiology: a sourcebook*. New York: Guilford Press.

Seligman, M. E. P., and Johnston, J. (1973). A cognitive theory of avoidance learning. In J. McGuigan and B. Lumsden (Eds.), *Contemporary approaches to conditioning and learning*. New York: Wiley.

Taylor, S. (1996). Meta-analysis of cognitive-behavioral treatments for social phobia. *Journal of Behavior Therapy and Experimental Psychiatry, 27*(1), 1-9.

Taylor, S. (2000). *Understanding and treating panic disorder. Cognitive-behavioral approaches*. Chichester: John Wiley and Sons.

Thompson, J. A., Charlton, P. F. C., Kerry, R., and Lee, D. (1995). An open trial of exposure therapy based on deconditioning for post-traumatic stress disorder. *British Journal of Clinical Psychology, 34*, 407-416.

van Oppen, P., de Haan, E., van Balkom, A. J., Spinhoven, P., Hoogduin, K., and van Dyck, R. (1995). Cognitive therapy and exposure in vivo in the treatment of obsessive compulsive disorder. *Behaviour Research and Therapy, 33*(4), 379-390.

White, J. R. (1999). *Overcoming generalized anxiety disorder - Client manual: a relaxation, cognitive restructuring, and exposure-based protocol for the treatment of GAD*. Oakland, CA: New Harbinger Publications.

World Health Organization. (1992). *The ICD-10 Classification of mental and behavioral disorders: diagnostic criteria for research*. Geneva: World Health Organization.

World Health Organization. (1993). *Composite International Diagnostic Interview - Version 1.1*. Geneva: World Health Organization.

In: Fear in Cognitive Neuroscience
Editor: Salvatore Campanella, pp. 157-178
ISBN: 1-59454-502-2

Chapter 7

FEAR EMOTIONAL EXPRESSION IN PSYCHOPATHY AND ANTISOCIAL PERSONALITY DISORDER

Laurent Servais[1], Edith Stillemans[1], Stephan De Smet[2], Bruno Piccinin[3], Pierre Fossion[4], Jérôme Laville[5], Pierre Titeca[1], Jacques Titeca[1] and Elsa Hoffmann[1]

[1]Centre Hospitalier Jean Titeca, Rue de la Luzerne, 11 – 1030 Bruxelles, Belgique.
[2]Hôpital Militaire Reine Astrid, Service de Psychiatrie – Bruxelles, Belgique.
[3]Institution Publique de Protection de la Jeunesse de Fraipont – Liège, Belgique.
[4]Centre Hospitalier Universitaire Brugmann,
Place Van Gehuchten, 4 – 1020 Bruxelles, Belgique.
[5]Centre Hospitalier Psychiatrique de Bordeaux, France.

INTRODUCTION: PSYCHOPATHY AND THE EMOTIONS

The brain's structure, function and development are the result of the interactions of several factors, including genetic, physiological and experiential variables. At the neurobiological level it has been well demonstrated that the quality of early interaction will determine the structure and wiring of the brain and, therefore, the cerebral functions as well.

As regards the cerebral functions involved in the emotions, the developmental neurosciences have demonstrated the importance of cooperative communication of infant-caregiver attachments for emotional and cognitive development. This gradual emotional and cognitive development is due in no small measure to social interactions in which attachment to the caregivers predominates in the early years of life, subsequently diversifying during infancy and adolescence.

Three stages in the development of the emotional functions can be distinguished. The acquisition of basic emotions (i.e. as inferred from the facial expressions) is the first stage of emotional development, and begins in the first year of life through the infant's early interactions with the mother figure, especially the infant's recognition of the facial expressions of the people in his surroundings in response to certain stimuli as well as the gestures of imitation (Bowlby, 1969).

Subsequently, at the end of the second year, more complex emotions such as shame, envy, guilt and embarrassment emerge (Gordon; in Kaplan and Sadock, 2000).

Finally, empathy – defined as the ability to perceive and, to a certain extent, to experience the emotional responses of others – appears soon afterwards and continues to develop throughout infancy. However, certain less structured and more rudimentary forms of empathy are also found from the age of one year (Gordon; in Kaplan and Sadock, 2000).

To sum up, emotional and cognitive development are inextricably linked. In particular, normal social functioning can only be established via social interactions of high quality in which the emotions act as the basic signals of social regulation. This means that the processing of emotional expressions is fundamental for normal socialisation and interaction.

These findings are of especial interest in the study of what one might call 'the psychopathic disorder', which can be conceptualised as a disability that disrupts the socialisation process. As regards the emotional functions of psychopathic subjects, there is growing agreement that the psychopathic disorder reflects a dysfunction in the systems that process socialisation due to fear conditioning. In other words: in psychopathic individuals, systems that mediate fear (and probably other emotions) are considered to be dysfunctional. From this point of view, psychopathic individuals form an interesting group in which to study the brain structures involved in moral and social reasoning and the emotional process.

This chapter is divided into two parts. First, the nosographical work that seeks to acquire a clearer view of the concept of psychopathy will be discussed both in the adult and in the infant and adolescent. Second, research into the neurophysiological, neurocognitive and neuroanatomical bases of psychopathy will be presented.

Part I: Nosology and Psychopathic Disorders

In this section, the taxonomic work that seeks to better delineate the psychopathological profiles associated with antisocial or asocial behaviour will be discussed, with an emphasis on the profiles' relationship to emotional disturbances. From a developmental perspective, the early manifestations of the psychopathic disorder in infancy and adolescence will also be dealt with.

A precise knowledge of the nosographical categories formulated to acquire a clearer picture of antisocial behaviour, such as the concept of psychopathy, will help us to understand the heterogeneous and sometimes divergent nature of the research findings for this population.

N.B.

Antisocial acts and criminality in general confront our post-modern societies with major challenges.

Decoding criminality and antisocial behaviour from a neurobiological, neurocognitive or psychopathological standpoint is only one way among many of understanding these complex phenomena. So as to avoid becoming embroiled in an enervating reductionism, one should bear in mind that the sociological and criminological points of view are also especially important. Any attempt to understand, prevent or counteract these forms of behaviour must seek to integrate the various existing frames of reference with a view to providing global and coherent responses to these phenomena.

Nonetheless, if one studies the phenomenon of delinquency in any sort of depth one discovers that, from a psychopathological perspective, only one subcategory of delinquency is ultimately ascribable to psychopathological conditions. This will, however, be an important one, because this subset comprises individuals who will persist in their criminal activities.

Moreover, this subcategory is especially important for society as a whole. In fact, in terms of human suffering the repercussions on the victims and their families of these antisocial forms of behaviour cannot be quantified, any more than those that affect the perpetrators themselves and their families. Quite apart from the high fiscal cost to which criminality gives rise (Scott et al, 2001), seeking coherent and ethical responses to this complex problem must be a priority for any society that wishes to consider itself to be democratic. Research in the cognitive sciences can contribute to an understanding of this challenge to society.

1. History and Definition of the Concept of Psychopathy

The sciences of modern psychiatry and criminology gradually emerged during the 19th century. They subsequently differentiated themselves as human sciences as part of a process that had actually begun during the Renaissance. Within this historical framework, in which the first nosographies of mental disturbances gradually saw the light of day, psychopathy as a clinical entity slowly acquired sharper definition alongside other no less important entities, such as melancholia or, later, schizophrenia.

At the very beginning of this process, Benjamin Rush (1786) first put forward the idea that *'moral behaviour is brain based'*. Shortly afterwards, Pinel (1801) described a syndrome characterised by 'blind impulses leading to acts of violence' without interference from the reasoning. He called it 'mania without delirium'. Shortly afterwards, his pupil Esquirol reformulated it as 'instinctive monomania'.

Later, various definitions aimed at more sharply characterising subjects involved in criminal conduct would follow, each reflecting the currently prevailing or fashionable psychological theories. Indeed, throughout history antisocial behaviour has often been considered from two opposing perspectives: as an internal deficit or as an ecological and adaptive response to extremely disrupted, violent and disorganised environments.

Schematically, the nosographical descriptions place the emphasis sometimes on social maladaptation, sometimes on unbalanced an unstable behaviour. In parallel with this, the concept of affective coldness (absence of feelings of guilt, absence of empathy, etc,) gradually emerged as a characteristic trait of psychopathic behaviour.

In 1941, Cleckley published the first edition of his 'Mask of Sanity'. In this standard reference work, the author isolated 16 characteristic traits, among which emotional disturbance is clearly identified. In this connection one can cite in particular lack of remorse or shame, lack of empathy, absence of nervousness, egocentricity and failure to form intimate attachments with others, failure to learn from punishment, and general impoverishment of major affective reactions. Referring to the gulf between the linguistic and the experiential components of emotion, Johns and Quay (1962) wrote that the psychopath knows the 'words' of emotion but not the music (in Patrick et al, 1993).

Shortly afterwards, in his 'Clinical Psychopathology', Kurt Schneider (1950) distinguished, among the different pathological personalities, 'cold psychopaths'[1]. As far as one knows, he was the first author to present affective coldness as a central trait of a personality disorder in which behavioural disturbances are also to be found. Schneider wrote: 'cold psychopaths are people for whom compassion, shame, honour, repentance and conscience simply do not exist... they are often impulsive, brutal and cruel in their actions'.

2. Categorical Nosographical Approaches

At the present time, the two most widely used definitions are the antisocial personality disorder (APD) of the Diagnostic and Statistical Manual (DSM IV) and the Hare Psychopathy CheckList Revised – PCL-R; 1991) (Hare, 1970; 1981; 1986; 1991; Harpur and Hare, 1994).

a) The Antisocial Personality Disorder

Among the criteria laid down for the antisocial personality disorder of the DSM-IV, which is characterised by a pervasive pattern of antisocial behaviour, the flattening of emotional expression is virtually absent. Only the final criterion makes any reference to the impoverishment of the emotional responses, while limiting them to an absence of guilt feelings and indifference to the consequences of the conduct leading up to an action. This diagnostic category, which is in fact almost solely based on behavioural aspects, does not take into account the global emotional impoverishment that characterises the behaviour of the psychopathic personality. In fact, the concept of psychopathy is, *stricto sensu*, distinct from but related to the antisocial personality disorder: impulsivity and antisocial behaviour alone are insufficient to define personalities that fit the construct of psychopathy.

b) Hare Psychopathy Checklist Revised

In the adult subject, the Hare Psychopathy CheckList Revised (PCL-R) is currently considered to be the most effective tool for establishing a diagnosis of psychopathy. The revised version, published in 1991, contains 20 precise, detailed and differentiated items that help identify the presence of the traits that are traditionally regarded as constituents of this syndrome. These items are scored from 0 to 2, and a total equal to or higher than the fixed cut-off of 30 is sufficient for a diagnosis of psychopathy according to PCL-R.

As regards the emotional problems described above, the PCL-R broadly takes these into account through the inclusion of items such as 'need for stimulation/proneness to boredom'

---

[1] Schneider uses the term 'psychopath' in its true etymological sense, i.e. to mean a personality disorder seen in terms of a deviation from the mean or normal condition, in contrast to the psychoses, which, for this author, correspond by virtue of their somatic basis to the criteria of an illness in its generally accepted sense.

(item 3), 'lack of remorse or guilt' (item 6), 'shallow affect' (item 7), 'callous/lack of empathy' (item 8).

The diagnosis of psychopathy as conceived by the Hare Psychopathy CheckList Revised therefore simultaneously takes into account antisocial behaviour and specific personality traits. From this point of view, factor analyses have made it possible to use the Hare Psychopathy CheckList Revised to isolate two principal factors (Cooke and Michie, 1997; Harpur, Hakstian and Hare, 1988). The first of these factors refers to personality traits, and is composed of the items 'glibness/superficial charm, grandiose senses of self worth, pathological lying, conning/manipulative, lack of remorse or guilt, shallow affect, callous/lack of empathy and failure to accept responsibility for own actions'. It is worth noting that, within this factor, two types of traits can be distinguished, namely traits associated with a problem of narcissism (glibness, superficial charm, grandiose sense of self worth, pathological lying, conning, manipulative) and traits that reflect a disturbance of the affectivity in the sense of deficiency of emotional experience (lack of remorse or guilt, shallow affect, callousness, lack of empathy, failure to accept responsibility for own actions). The second might be considered as an antisocial behaviour factor defined largely by instrumental aggression, which is highly characteristic of psychopathic individuals (Woodworth et al, 2002) and the committing of a wide range of offences. It comprises the items 'need for stimulation/proneness to boredom, parasitic lifestyle, poor behavioural control, early behaviour problems, lack of realistic long-term goals, impulsivity, irresponsibility, juvenile delinquency and revocation of conditional release'.

C. Commentary

The relationship between psychopathy according to the PCL-R criteria and the antisocial personality disorder is asymmetric, since the PCL-R criteria include an assessment of antisocial forms of behaviour as well as personality traits. Predictably, high scores on the second factor are strongly associated with the diagnosis of APD, while high scores on the first factor are less strongly associated. The PCL-R diagnosis is more specific for a subcategory of APD: about 90% of psychopathic offenders meet APD criteria, but only about 25% of those diagnosed with APD meet the PCL-R criteria for psychopathy.

Moreover, whereas scores on the second factor decline with age, scores on the first do not. This stability might reflect the fact that emotional deficit is one of the central features of psychopathy, related to neurocognitive impairment (see below).

3. Dimensional Nosographical Approaches

In a manner complementary to the central definition of psychopathy according to the DSM IV and Hare, other writers have put forward dimensional models rather than categorical ones in their investigation of personality disorders.

Cloninger and Svrakic (1997), for example, suggest that the antisocial personality is characterised by a specific triad, with a high score on the dimension 'novelty seeking' (i.e. the tendency to respond to new stimuli with excitement or exaltation, curiosity, impulsiveness, non-conformism, etc.), a low score on the dimension 'harm avoidance' (i.e. the tendency to respond in a relatively uninvolved manner to aversive stimuli, absence of timidity, pessimism, anxiety, etc.) and a low score on the dimension 'reward dependence' (i.e. the tendency to respond weakly to signals of social and interpersonal gratification, absence of sensitivity, etc.) (Cannon et al, 1993; Cloninger et al, 1995; Sigvardson et al, 1996; Compton et al, 1996; Schmidt et al, 1996; in Pélissolo et al, 1997).

4. Psychopathy as a Developmental Disorder

Psychopathy and antisocial personality disorder are considered to be severe developmental disorders. Many studies, both retrospective (Loeber, 1982, 1990, 1991, 2002) and prospective (Stevenson and Goodman, 2001; Harrington, 2001; Raine, 1996; Caspi, 1996), have shed light on the links between behavioural problems during infancy and adolescence (in particular problems of conduct) and antisocial personality disorder, psychopathy and criminality in adulthood, the first being a very powerful predictor of the second. In parallel with this, confronted with the low level of effectiveness associated with therapeutic approaches to dealing with adult antisocial offenders, more attention has been focused on their early identification in the hope of making effective early interventions and establishing successful prevention programs.

Behavioural problems in infants and adolescents, such as impulsive, oppositional or transgressive behaviour, are, according to the DSM-IV, represented in three different syndromes: the Attention-Deficit Hyperactivity Disorder (ADHD), the Oppositional Defiant Disorder (ODD) and the Conduct Disorder (CD). In parallel, several child and adolescent psychopathy inventories have recently been developed, such as the Psychopathy Screening Device (Frick and Hare, 2001) and the Childhood Psychopathy Scale (Lynam, 1997).

A. CD

A.1. Clinical Features

Clinically, Conduct Disorder (CD) refers to the clustering of persistent antisocial acts of children and adolescents. The symptoms are clustered in four groups: aggression to people and animals, destruction of property, deceitfulness and theft, and, finally, serious violation of rules. All these symptoms with just one exception ('often lies to obtain goods or favours or to avoid obligations' (i.e., 'cons' others') item 11) are descriptions of transgressive behaviour forms. In a manner that is somewhat congruent with that of the APD, the subject's psychological functioning, including the emotional register, is passed over. The absence of a sense of guilt and, more generally, emotional coldness, do not form part of the diagnostic criteria of this problem, any more than does the constant tendency among these subjects to project onto the world around them the blame for their behavioural peculiarities (projection or external attribution). As a result, this quite aspecific diagnosis covers a very wide range of problems.

To sum up: conduct disorder is a heterogeneous problem that 'can best be described as a final common pathway for several initially divergent developmental trajectories' (Steiner, in Kaplan and Sadock, 2000).

A.2. Etiological Factors

From an etiological perspective, twins and adoption studies indicate a large shared environmental (familial) effect, a moderate non-shared environmental effect and a modest genetic effect.

Adoption studies suggest that an interaction between genetic vulnerability and unfavourable family conditions. The importance of the role played by the latter in the genesis of CD is today widely accepted and documented (see introduction). Briefly, poor parenting, rejection of the child, abusive and neglectful behaviour, child maltreatment and parental disharmony with or without violence are obvious risk factors for the development of conduct disorder.

At the neurobiological level, as demonstrated experimentally in the sensory and motors areas, experience plays a fundamental role in the modulation of the synaptic connectivity of areas of emotional and cognitive association. These data are in accordance with the fact that an individual's lifelong emotional abilities reflect an internal representation of the reactions of caregivers in the first years of life.

A.3. Psychopathy Construct in Youth: Callous-Unemotional Traits

The link between conduct disorder in adolescence and the antisocial personality in adulthood has been demonstrated by numerous prospective and retrospective studies. Recently, in a prospective study, J Kim-Cohen et al (2003) confirmed once again that CD (and ODD) are precursors of antisocial personality disorder. Even so, in this study the aspecific and heterogeneous character of CD is underlined by the fact that this diagnosis is also over-represented in the precursors of the main psychiatric adult disorders (anxiety disorder, depression, schizophreniform disorders, eating disorders and mania).

Confronted with the relatively aspecific character of CD as a predictor of APD or psychopathy, some writers, such as PJ Frick and colleagues, have reassigned a central position to affective disturbances, including emotional coldness. In 1994, in a factor analysis of a measure of psychopathy in a sample of 95 clinic-referred children between the ages of 6 and 13, these authors found two dimensions of psychopathic behaviour: one associated with impulsivity and conduct problems (I/CP) and the other associated with the interpersonal and motivational aspects of psychopathy, called callous/unemotional (CU). Scores derived from the CU factor were only moderately associated with measures of conduct problems, and exhibited a different pattern of associations on several criteria that have been associated with psychopathy (e.g., sensation seeking) or childhood antisocial behaviour (e.g., low intelligence, poor school achievement, and anxiety). For these authors, their results suggest that, in youth, psychopathic personality features and conduct problems are independent. In the same way, a one-year follow-up study (Frick et al, 2003) shows that callous-unemotional (CU) traits are predictive of conduct problem severity, severity and type of aggression and self-reported delinquency. In a study of adjudicated youths, these traits, in contrast to behavioural factors (i.e., impulsivity/conduct problems), were also found to be associated with lower emotional distress and a specific social information-processing pattern characterised by an increased focus on the positive aspects of aggression and a decreased focus on the negative aspects of hostile acts (Pardini et al, 2003). This study reinforced the hypothesis of the two-dimensional nature of psychopathy in youths.

Furthermore, a study of juvenile delinquents by Christian et al (1997) found that children with CU traits had more conduct problems with a greater diversity, a stronger history of police contacts, and more familial antecedents of antisocial personality disorder. So, for these authors, CU traits with significant conduct problems seem to designate a subgroup with a very severe pattern of antisocial behaviour who correspond more closely to adult psychopathy.

Finally, Loeber et al (2002) recently published a study about psychopathology antecedents in a clinic-referred sample of young males. These authors found that the best predictors of APD were callous/unemotional behaviour, depression and marijuana use.

B. ODD

B.1. Clinical Features

The central feature of ODD is a recurrent pattern of negativistic, defiant, disobedient and hostile behaviour towards authority figures, which persists for at least six months. The conduct leading up to the heteroaggressive physical act does not form part of the diagnostic criteria for this problem (APA, DSM IV). The subject's provocations and transgressions, even if they do affect his functioning from a social, scholastic or professional point of view, are not sufficiently serious to warrant a reaction from the law enforcement agencies.

B.2. Etiological Factors

The etiological studies of ODD are usually to be found in the body of research on conduct disorder. Briefly, etiological factors of ODD are, like CD, multifactorial (genetic, familial and environmental).

B.3. Psychopathy Construct in Youth

The link between this disorder and the antisocial personality or psychopathy remains unclear and contradictory. The remarks made above regarding CD as a relatively unspecific predictor of problems in adulthood (i.e., psychopathy) are even truer of ODD and could at least partially explain the contradictory data encountered in the literature.

C. ADHD

C.1. Clinical Features

Children with ADHD display early symptoms of hyperactivity, inattention and impulsive behaviour.

C.2. Etiological Factors

It has been consistently observed that ADHD and CD frequently co-occur.

Numerous findings indicate that CD and ADHD share a common genetic aetiology, but that ADHD + CD is a genetically and clinically more severe variant of ADHD alone (Thapar et al, 2001). Clinical prospective studies have largely confirmed that ADHD+CD is a high risk for a worse outcome and that ADHD alone is a low risk for progression to antisocial disorders. For Lynam (1996, 1998), the group of children with the comorbid condition ADHD+CD contains the future psychopathic adult.

C.3. Psychopathy Construct in Youth

From the perspective of the emotions, Barry et al (2000) found that children with both ADHD and a conduct problem diagnosis (ODD or CD) displayed features typically associated with psychopathy, such as a lack of fearfulness and a reward-dominant response style, all the more so when they displayed callous-unemotional traits.

This problem could therefore only have a clear association with APD or psychopathy when it is associated with CD and when the predominant symptomatology is impulsiveness.

PART II: NEUROPSYCHOLOGICAL, NEUROPHYSIOLOGICAL, NEUROCOGNITIVE AND NEUROANATOMICAL BASES

Many studies have sought to shed light on the biological bases of behaviour and antisocial personality disorder. To this end, neurocognitive investigations, evaluations of the functioning of the autonomous nervous system and cerebral imagery (both structural and functional) have been utilised. A synthesis of the relevant data from the literature is presented in this section.

1. Neuropsychological Measures and Antisocial Behaviour

It has been known for some considerable time that frontal lobe damage is associated with emotional and behavioural changes, such as irresponsibility and difficulty in tolerating frustration, frequent impulsivity and increased levels of aggression, shallow affect, lack of empathy and lack of concern for social rules. To some extent, these clinical features mimic the antisocial personality disorder. The term 'acquired sociopathy' was introduced for those individuals who, after lesions of the orbitofrontal (ventral) and medial frontal cortex, presented DSM-III diagnostic criteria for 'sociopathic disorder' (Damasio, 1994). These criteria included 'defective planning', 'lack of remorse' and 'being reckless regarding others' personal safety'. In parallel, the hypothesis was formulated that developmental psychopathy could at least partially be explained by a dysfunction of these cerebral structures.

A. Executive Functions

The literature on neuropsychological measures of executive functions in psychopathic or antisocial disorders is unclear and contradictory. Various factors can explain this confusion:

1. variation in diagnostic criteria (PCL R vs. APD) ;
2. selection bias associated, for example, with the method of recruitment (samples derived from psychiatric hospital, prisons, forensic settings or community) ;

3. absence of screening for psychiatric comorbidity, such as substance abuse or psychotic disorders;
4. variation in the inclusion of healthy control comparison groups or, when this is the case, comparison with poorly matched healthy control groups;
5. use of a variety of neuropsychological tasks could have contributed to these conflicting findings.

Thus, Hare (1984) found no evidence of executive function deficits in psychopathic criminals compared with non-psychopathic criminals.

However, in a recent meta-analytic review of 39 studies, Morgan and Lilienfeld (2000) concluded that there was a significant link between executive function deficits and antisocial personality disorder. They also concluded that APD was associated with a broader executive function deficit than was psychopathy.

Dinn and Harris (2000) support the view that a selective orbitofrontal deficit may be associated with psychopathy, as do Lapierre et al (1995), who showed that incarcerated psychopathic subjects were significantly impaired on tasks considered sensitive to orbitofrontal/ventromedial-prefrontal function, including a visual go/no-go discrimination task, Porteus Maze Test and an odour identification task, in comparison with matched control subjects (non-psychopathic inmates). These authors also found that psychopathic subjects did not display performance deficits on measures sensitive to dorsolateral-prefrontal and posterorolandic function.

For Dinn and Harris (2000), the executive function deficits (i.e., dorsolateral) among psychopathic subjects are associated with comorbid psychiatric conditions, while the core interpersonal and affective characteristics associated with psychopathy (egocentricity, callousness, manipulativeness, guile, lack of empathy and remorse) may result from orbitofrontal dysfunction.

More recently, Dolan (2002) found both orbitofrontal and dorsolateral deficits when comparing subjects with APD to healthy controls matched only for age and IQ. In this study, comorbid psychiatric conditions such as psychosis, substance abuse or personality disorders were well controlled.

Further researches are needed to arrive at definitive conclusions. These studies should take into account all the potential biases and limitations described above.

Among infants and adolescents, publications are few and far between and are again contradictory (Raine, 2002a, 2002b; Dery, 1999; Giancola, 1996, 2001; Lahey, 1995; Stevens, 2003).

B. Emotional Processing

Several studies have shown that psychopathic traits are associated with abnormalities in the processing of emotional stimuli.

From an experimental viewpoint, these studies have primarily investigated the ability of psychopathic subjects to recognise and/or identify facial expressions of emotion or tones of voice.

The results show, both in adult subjects (Kosson, 2002; Blair, 2002) and in children (Loney, 2003; Blair, 2001; Stevens, 2001), that subjects with psychopathic traits exhibit deficits in the processing of emotional stimuli, in particular sadness and fear.

2. Psychophysiological Measures and Antisocial Behaviour

Introduction

The psychophysiological measures usually include the electrodermal response, the modulation of the startle reflex and the electromyographic activity of the corrugator muscle.

Schematically, the electrodermal activity is considered as an indicator of emotion arousal though the modulation of the startle reflex as an index of emotional valence. According to Lang (1985; in Patrick, 1993), 'emotional responses to stimuli are defined in terms of two orthogonal dimensions: affective valence and arousal. Valence refers to the directionality of the elicited action disposition, varying from avoidance to approach; arousal refers to the intensity of activation of the response'.

Finally, the measures of the electromyographic activity of the corrugator muscle are regarded as an index of emotional expression.

Adult Studies

From the 1960s onwards, studies have focused on the autonomic nervous responses of psychopathic individuals in punishing and threatening situations.

Several psychophysiological studies have repeatedly found a low autonomic responsiveness in psychopaths with reduced electrodermal responses during anticipation of aversive stimuli related to feelings of fear or threat (Arnett et al, 1997, Hare, 1978, Arnett, 1997; in Herpertz, 2001), or during processing of fearful facial expressions.

Several studies have also shown the same deficit to sad expressions in psychopathic individuals compared with controls (House and Milligan, 1976, Aniskiewicz, 1979, Chaplin et al, 1995, Blair et al, 1997; in Blair et al, 1999).

In a major study, Patrick et al (1993) showed that in psychopaths the startle eye reflex did not show a larger and faster blink during unpleasant visual stimuli than during pleasant stimuli. This impairment of the startle reflex is correlated with a high score in the PCL-R factor 1 (i.e. personality traits). Patrick concluded that 'emotional detachment – defined by factor 1 in PCL-R – appears to be the factor most pertinent to psychopaths'.

These results support the hypothesis that in psychopathic individuals there is a deficit in brain structures governing negative affects (i.e., the amygdala).

Recently, Herpertz et al (2001) used multiple psychophysiological measures (electrodermal response, modulation of the startle reflex, electromyographic activity of the corrugator muscle) to compare emotional responses to pleasant and unpleasant stimuli between criminal offenders with psychopathy or with borderline personality disorder and controls.

The results once again supported the theory that psychopaths display a lack of fear in response to aversive stimuli but also a general deficit in processing affective information whether the stimuli are positive or negative. In contrast to Patrick's results, psychopaths showed no modulation of the startle response in relation to any kind of emotional stimulus. Furthermore, the corrugator muscle response of psychopaths suggested rare aversive facial expressions. The authors add that, although all the psychophysiological data suggest emotional hyporesponsiveness, psychopaths' self-reports of their emotional responses did not reflect this deficiency. This dissociation between self-report and physiological data is paralleled by other studies showing dissociation between the linguistic and experiential components of emotion in psychopaths.

In the same way, Patrick et al (1994) studied low- and high-psychopathic individuals while they imagined fearful and neutral scenes in a cued sentence-processing task. As expected, subjects with a high level of psychopathy showed fewer physiological reactions during fearful imagery, in accordance with the theory of dissociation between semantic and emotional processes in psychopathy.

Youth Studies

Some findings in youth suggest that these deficits (i.e., autonomic arousal or reactivity) appear before adulthood.

For instance, Raine et al (1995), in a 14-year prospective study, found that high levels of autonomic arousal and orientation at age 15 were protective against the development of criminal behaviour at age 29.

Herpetz et al (2001) studied autonomic arousal and electrodermal responses to orienting and aversive stimuli in boys aged 8 to 13 years with Attention Deficit Hyperactivity Disorder (ADHD) + Conduct Disorder (CD) or ADHD alone. As expected, in boys with the comorbid condition they found a decrement of autonomic responses and a faster habituation to orienting and aversive startling stimuli compared with children with ADHD alone. In short, boys with ADHD+CD, who are at high risk for psychopathic evolution, displayed a psychophysiological response pattern very similar to that reported in adult psychopaths.

Psychophysiological Abnormalities as a Sign of Structural Dysfunctions

Like the hypothalamus and limbic system, which are crucial components of the neural circuitry regulating emotions and autonomic functions, the orbitofrontal system also contributes to the regulation of autonomic nervous system activity, including electrodermal activity and the rapid control of arterial pressure (Damasio et al, 1990, Guyton, 1991, Tranel and Damasio, 1994, Tranel et al, 1988; in Dinn and Harris, 2000; Herpertz et al, 2001). Bilateral orbitofrontal lesions in human subjects induce fewer reactive electrodermal responses during exposure to emotionally charged stimuli (Tranel et al, 1988; in Dinn and Harris, 2000). Moreover, patients with amygdala lesions show impoverished aversive conditioning and reduced augmented startle reflexes similar to those seen in psychopaths (Hare et al, 1978, Davis, 1986, Patrick et al, 1993, Bechara et al, 1995, LaBar et al, 1995, Angrilli et al, 1996, LeDoux, 1998; in Blair et al, 1999).

These conclusions among patients with specific cerebral lesions underline the importance of these structures in the autonomic relationships associated with the processing of emotional information.

3. Neuroimaging and Antisocial Behaviour

A. The Cerebral Structures Involved in Emotional Responses: The Supremacy of the Amygdala

There is reasonable agreement concerning the anatomical structure involved in processing expressions of fear, in which the amygdala plays a central role.

This structure, which is a part of the limbic system, displays an extremely complex connectivity with the rest of the brain and is considered as an alarm system when triggered by fear. Anatomically, the amygdala projects to most major areas of the brain: the hypothalamus (release of corticotrophin-releasing hormone – mobilisation of the fight-or-flight reaction), corpus striatum (system of movement), the cingulate, temporal and prefrontal cortices, the locus ceruleus (norepinephrine neurons, which in their turn project to the cortex, the brainstem and the limbic system), the brainstem and medulla (via the nearby central nucleus – autonomic nervous system). The amygdala, like the nearby hippocampus, receives projections from the thalamus and the temporal, insular, limbic and prefrontal cortices.

Briefly, when triggered by fear the amygdala stimulates the locus ceruleus activity to increase the reactivity of key brain areas and signals the brainstem to fix the face in a fearful expression and initiate autonomic reactions. Furthermore, the direct circuitry between amygdala and thalamus enables the amygdala to act as a repository for partly unconscious emotional impressions and memories. The circuitry between the amygdala, the hippocampus and the prefrontal cortex improves attention and mobilises a wide range of cognitive functions.

It is implicated in fear conditioning, which is recognised as a *sine qua non* for effective socialisation. The amygdala also plays an important role in the modulation of aggressive or submissive behaviours.

Moreover, the amygdala and the limbic system as a whole are highly interconnected with the prefrontal cortex. This is especially highly developed in humans and accounts for 29% of the entire neocortex[2]. As the work of Changeux J-P has underlined, it plays an essential part in the memory functions (especially in the working memory, i.e. the capacity to retain information during a task), the ability to verify the relevance of this information during a learning process and the ability to retain in the mind the objective to be reached during this learning process, deductive reasoning, and the imagination. It also makes it possible to understand the states of mind both of other people and of oneself.

To summarise, the various functions of the cortex are: attention span, perseverance, planning, judgement, impulse control, organisation, self-monitoring and supervision, problem solving, critical thinking, forward thinking, learning from experience and mistakes, ability to feel and express emotions, influencing of the limbic system, empathy, internal supervision.

B. Psychopathy and Structural Imagery

Raine (2000) compared prefrontal grey and white matter volumes using structural magnetic resonance imaging in 21 men with APD, 34 controls, 27 men with substance dependence and 21 psychiatric controls. The APD group showed a subtle structural deficit in the prefrontal grey matter cortex. Indeed, the APD subjects had an 11% reduction in prefrontal grey matter compared with a control group, a 14% reduction compared with a

[2] By way of comparison, in the chimpanzee it accounts for 17% of the whole of the neocortex.

substance-dependent group, and a 14% reduction compared with a psychiatric control group. These results establish for the first time the presence of this kind of structural deficit in APD subjects in a study where confounding factors (i.e., psychiatric comorbidity, psychoactive substance dependence, psychosocial factors) are well controlled.

A second study, by Woerman et al (2000), found significant frontal grey matter reduction, especially in the left anterior frontolateral cortex, in patients with temporal lobe epilepsy with recurrent episodic aggression. These patients were compared with normal controls and non-aggressive patients with the same pathology.

Reductions in the dorsal hippocampal volumes were also found in psychopaths (Laakso et al, 2001), in accordance with experimental results indicating the importance of the dorsal hippocampus in the acquisition of conditioned fear. These data reinforced theories that proposed that 'central features in the birth of psychopathy are due to a deficit in the acquisition of conditioned fear'.

C. Psychopathy and Functional Anatomy

In normal subjects, Blair et al (1999) found that neural response to sad and fearful facial expressions had in common left amygdala activation while angry expressions activated the right orbitofrontal cortex. They postulated that there are at least two systems that are implicated in response to different classes of aversive stimuli: the fear- and sad-related system involved in (social) aversive conditioning and the angry-related system that encourages behavioural extinction.

These data reinforced the hypothesis of a dysfunction of the amygdala in psychopathic individuals, since they suggest a selectively reduced autonomic response to fearful and sad expressions.

While several studies have emphasised a selectively reduced autonomic response to sad expressions, there is a limited number of functional neuroimaging studies in APD, psychopaths or violent offenders.

Raine (1994, 1998) found a decreased activation in prefrontal regions (and, more particularly, in the ventromedial regions) in murderers compared with healthy controls matched for age and sex during an auditory activation task. These authors also show that this reduction was primarily manifested in murderers without a history of psychosocial deprivation, suggesting that these deficits could best be explained by genetic rather than environmental influences.

Functional response to neutral and emotional words during a lexical decision task were studied by Intrator et al (1997) using a single photon emission computed tomography in psychopathic and non-psychopathic substance abusers and in community controls. Psychopathic subjects displayed greater relative activation in emotional rather than neutral conditions than the two non-psychopathic groups. This greater activation was interpreted as a reflection of the difficulties in processing emotional information. Furthermore, psychopaths activated more posterior brain regions, suggesting that processing semantic and affective information drew upon an atypical circuitry.

Schneider et al (2000), using an aversive classical conditioning paradigm, found differential effects in the amygdala and in the dorsolateral prefrontal cortex activation. Unexpectedly, psychopaths showed an overactivation of these regions, suggesting a need for an additional effort to form negative emotional associations.

During an affective memory task, functional magnetic resonance imaging (fMRI) of criminal psychopaths compared with criminal non-psychopaths and control subjects revealed a less affect-related activity in limbic structures and an overactivation in the bilateral frontotemporal cortex (Kiehl, 2001)

In a recent functional magnetic imaging study, Muller et al (2003) investigated 6 psychopaths and 6 controls to study the influence of positive and negative affective contents on brain activity. In this design, series of negative and positive pictures were shown while functional imaging was performed. This was of particular interest because this design did not demand the involvement of the higher cortical functions (e.g., attention, language, memory). For the two categories of stimuli, the results displayed multiple differences in hyper- or hypoactivation of the cortical and subcortical structures involved in emotion processing. These results reinforce the hypothesis of a dysfunction of the emotion-related cerebral networks in psychopathy.

Veit et al (2002) compared 4 psychopaths, 4 social phobics (characterised by excessive fear) and 7 healthy controls in differential aversive delay conditioning, with neutral faces as conditioned stimuli and painful pressure as unconditioned stimuli. Functional magnetic resonance imaging revealed brief amygdala activation in psychopaths. In contrast, healthy controls and moreover social phobics displayed differential activation in the limbic-prefrontal circuit (amygdala, anterior cingulate, insula, orbitofrontal cortex).

Neurofunctional imagery sometimes suggested activation deficits, and at other times overactivation of certain cerebral regions involved in the processing of emotional information. In particular, the amygdala displayed variations of this kind depending on the design used, especially according to the stimulation paradigm (e.g., recourse to a memory task or a direct stimulation).

Among psychopathic subjects, different activation patterns were revealed during the processing of positive or negative emotional stimuli.

Abnormal activation patterns have been found in different regions of the emotion-related brain circuit in psychopaths compared with healthy controls. To summarise, there is growing evidence of a disturbed interaction between top-down modulation, in which prefrontal regions play a key role, and bottom-up regulation where the role of the limbic system is central. The neurobiological underpinnings in psychopathy are evidence of a deregulation and a disturbed functional connectivity of the emotion-related area of the brain.

Conclusion

The psychopathologic definition of antisocial and psychopathic disorders calls for an improvement in the nosographical frameworks.

The definition of clinical syndromes constructed from behavioural descriptions (e.g. antisocial personality disorder) cover too varied and heterogeneous psychopathologic problems. This lack of specificity is not surprising when one notes that the antisocial behaviours very generally describe any action which transgresses the rules for living in society, in particular legislation, where no act, even an extremely serious one like homicide, is any indicator by itself of any individual psychology.

This non-specificity of antisocial behaviour is even more marked during childhood and adolescence (in children, antisocial acts are overwhelmingly defined by the transgression of family rules) where transgressive behaviours can be the expression of very varied difficulties, underlying irregular or oppositional psychological issues. Recent work indicates that behavioural problems are significantly found among precursors to many psychiatric pathologies in adulthood which again illustrates that the diagnosis of behavioural problems is very unspecific or even aspecific to any subsequent psychopathologic development.

Therefore, from a psychopathological point of view, antisocial behaviours, in addition to their repetitive and diverse nature, must correspond to certain precise criteria assessed by detailed analysis of their modus operandi and contextual elements of committing the act (systematic or non-systematic use of psychoactive substances, transgressions committed alone or in a group etc.). For example, the distinction between planned and unplanned antisocial acts needs to be integrated in a completely non-exhaustive manner into the evaluation of subjects deemed to be psychopaths. Impulsive aggressiveness must be distinguished from actions planned in cold blood.

In addition to antisocial behaviour, from a diagnostic perspective, the assessment of psychological function remains the most sensitive and most specific approach. In particular, emotional coldness is the key element which characterises the psychology of a psychopath. A certain number of other traits can be associated with this coldness as characteristics of this problem. For example, the absence of empathy can be understood as an expression of coldness. It is not actually possible to emotionally identify oneself with others and therefore it is not possible to even partly experience what the other party feels from their own emotional experience even slightly and differently. Likewise, how can the subject experience the feeling of guilt without being capable of experiencing the basic emotions of fear and sadness? In addition to this basic dimension, other specific dimensions are also present and integrated into the diagnostic assessment of the psychopathy, in particular narcissism.

In addition to these behavioural and psychopathological aspects, other parameters must be taken into consideration. For example, it must be possible to take into account the general functioning of subjects described as psychopathic (successful vs. unsuccessful). Similarly, it would be interesting to take into account the latent biographical aspects by making a distinction between psychopathic subjects who encountered major problems during early childhood (physical and sexual abuse, negligence, abandonment, problems in relationships, etc.) and those who experienced few if any early traumas, while controlling for the factors that are experimentally and clinically acknowledged to be risk factors in antisocial behaviour (neonatal problems (Raine, 1996), tobacco abuse during pregnancy (Wachslag, 1997), etc.).

From a neurocognitive, psychophysiological or anatomofunctional perspective, it is increasingly obvious that different parts of the neural network involved in emotion processing are disturbed in psychopathy.

Even if the neurocognitive evaluations remain heterogeneous and contradictory, the data produced by psychophysiological research and investigations of anatomofunctional imagery have revealed several dysfunctions or abnormal patterns. However contradictory the results of this research may be, it has contributed arguments to the two principal explanatory models of developmental psychopathy.

Indeed, the theory of acquired sociopathy proposed by Damasio (1994) implies an impairment in a somatic marker system as the cause of the aberrant social behaviour. This system is, in fact, the link between the subject's internal representations and a somatic marker, i.e. an autonomic nervous system response. These somatic markers are involved in the decision-making processes (the attention paid to the negative consequences to which an action could lead, and the alarm system).

So, according to this theory, psychopathic subjects suffer from a deficit in decision-making that reflects an inability to activate somatic states associated with the anticipation of rewards and punishments.

The theory of VIM (violence inhibition mechanism (Blair, 1995)) suggests that amygdala dysfunction is the main neural substrate involved in emotional deficits in psychopathic subjects. According to this theory, psychopaths fail to display the submission cues that normally inhibit aggressive responses, and this leads to impairments in empathy.

Alongside these models, which implicitly (and, indeed, explicitly) postulate a structural deficit or a deficit in functioning in certain cerebral regions, sight must not be lost of the fact that developmental psychopathy can also be seen as a mechanism of adaptation to especially unpleasant conditions of everyday life. Affective coldness could, in family environments in which extreme violence prevails, constitute the sole means of psychological survival in the child who, one must recall, cannot escape the family system in which he or she is growing up. From this perspective, the results of functional imagery research showing atypical overactivation of certain cerebral regions could reinforce the hypothesis of an adaptative mechanism of this kind.

Hence, it is apparent just how much the early diagnosis of psycho-affective development of children should be made a priority for the authorities when establishing major screening. In the same manner, setting up prevention programmes targeting families and children who display early cognitive or emotional difficulties is extremely important. This preventive approach is probably the only effective way of solving the problems of antisocial behaviour (Scott, 2001), since it is obvious that from adolescence onwards – and even more so in adulthood – therapeutic interventions have a very limited impact.

BIBLIOGRAPHY

Barry CT., Frick PJ., DeShaso TM., McCoy MG., Ellis M., Loney BR., The importance of callous-unemotional traits for extending the concept of psychopathy to children, *J. Abnorm. Psychol.*, 2000; 109(2): 335-40.

Blair R.J., A cognitive developmental approach to mortality: investigating the psychopath, *Cognition,* 1995; 57(1): 1-29.

Blair R.J.R., Neurocognitive models of aggression, the antisocial personality disorders, and psychopathy, *J. Neurol. Neurosurg. Psychiatry,* 2001, 71: 727-731.

Blair R.J.R., Cipolotti L., Impaired social response reversal, a case of 'acquired sociopathy', *Brain,* 2000, 123: 1122-1141.

Blair RJ, Colledge E, Murray L, Mitchell DG, A selective impairment in the processing of sad and fearful expressions in children with psychopathic tendencies, *J. Abnorm. Child. Psychol,* 2001, 29(6): 491-8.

Blair RJ., Mitchell DG., Richell RA., Kelly S., Leonard A., Newman C., Scott SK., Turning a deaf ear to fear: impaired recognition of vocal affect in psychopathic individuals, *J. Abnorm. Psychol.,* 2002; 111(4): 682-6.

Blair R.J.R., Morris J.S., Frith C.D., Perrett D.I., Dolan R.J., *Dissociable neural responses to facial expressions of sadness and anger,* Oxford University Press, 1999.

Bowlby J., Attachment and loss: Attachment, vol 1. *Basic books*, New York, 1969.

Brower M.C., Price B.H., Neuropsychiatry of frontal lobe dysfunction in violent and criminal behaviour: a critical review, *J. Neurol. Neurosurg. Psychiatry,* 2001, 71: 720-726.

Caspi A., Moffitt T.E., Newman D.L., Silva P.A., Behavioral observations at age 3 years predict adult psychiatric disorders. Longitudinal evidence from a birth cohort, *Arch. Gen. Psychiatry,* 1996; 53(11): 1033-9.

Changeux J-P, L'homme de vérité, Ed. *Odile Jacob*, 2002.

Christian RE., Frick PJ., Hill NL., Tyler L., Frazer DR., Psychopathy and conduct problems in children: II. Implications for subtyping children with conduct problems, *J. Am. Acad. Child Adolesc Psychiatry,* 1997; 36(2): 233-41.

Cleckley H, 1982, The Mask of Sanity (rev. Ed.), St. Louis, MO: C.V. *Mosby* (published 1941).

Cloninger C.R., Svrakic D.M., Integrative psychobiological approach to psychiatric assessment and treatment, *Psychiatry,* 1997; 60(2): 120-41.

Cooke D.J., Michie C., Refining the construct of psychopathy: towards a hierarchical model, *Psychol. Assess,* 2001; 13(2): 171-88.

Cooke D.J., Michie C., Psychopathy across cultures: North America and Scotland compared, *J. Abnorm. Psychol,* 1999; 108(1): 58-68.

Damasio AR, Descartes' error: emotion, reason and the human brain. New York, Putnam, 1994.

Dery M., Toupin J., Pauze R., Mercier H., Fortin L., Neuropsychological characteristics of adolescents with conduct disorder: association with attention-deficit hyperactivity and aggression, *J. Abnorm. Child. Psychol,* 1999; 27(3): 225-36.

Dinn W., Harris C., Neurocognitive function in antisocial personality disorder, *Psychiatry Research,* 2000 ; 97: 173-190.

Dolan M., What neuroimaging tells us about psychopathic disorders, Symposium on brain imaging, *Hospital Medicine,* 2002, 63, 6.

Esquirol J. E. D., Des Maladies Mentales considérées sous les Rapports Médical, Hygiénique et Médico-Légal, Paris: *J.B. Baillière,* 1838.

Farrington DP, Ohlin LE, Wilson JQ, Understanding and controlling crime: *Toward a new research strategy.* New York: Springer-Verlag, 1986.

Frick PJ., Cornell AH., Barry CT., Bodin SD., Dane HE., Callous-unemotional traits and conduct problems in the prediction of conduct problem severity, aggression, and self-report of delinquency, *J. Abnorm. Child. Psychol.,* 2003; 31(4): 457-70.

Frick, P.J. and Hare, R.D., The Antisocial Process Screening Device (APSD), 2001, Toronto: *Multi-Health Systems.*

Frick PJ., O'Brien BS., Wootton JM., McBurnett K., Psychopathy and conduct problems in children, *J. Abnorm. Psychol.,* 1994; 103(4): 700-7.

Giancola P.R., Martin C.S., Tarter R.E., Pelham W.E., Moss H.B., Executive cognitive functioning and aggressive behavior in preadolescent boys at high risk for substance abuse/dependence, *J. Stud. Alcohol,* 1996; 57(4): 352-9.

Giancola P.R., Moss H.B., Martin C.S., Kirisci L., Tarter R.E., Executive cognitive functioning predicts reactive aggression in boys at high risk or substance abuse: a prospective study, *Alcohol. Clin. Exp. Res,* 1996; 20(4): 740-4.

Giancola PR, Parker AM., A six-year prospective study of pathways toward drug use in adolescent boys with and without a family history of a substance use disorder., *J. Stud. Alcohol.* 2001 Mar;62(2):166-78.

Hare RD, Performance of psychopaths on cognitive tasks related to frontal lobe function, *J. Abnorm. Psychol,* 1984; 93: 133-140.

Hare R.D., The Hare Psychopathy Checklist-Revised manual, *Multi-Health System,* 1991.

Hare RD, Thorvaldson SA, Psychopathy and response to electrical stimulation, *J. Abnorm. Psychol.* 1970 Dec;76(3):370-4.

Harpur TJ, Hakstian AR, Hare RD., Factor structure of the Psychopathy Checklist., *J. Consult. Clin. Psychol.* 1988 Oct;56(5):741-7.

Harpur TJ, Hare RD., Assessment of psychopathy as a function of age, *J. Abnorm. Psychol.* 1994 Nov;103(4):604-9.

Harrington R., Developmental continuities and discontinuities, *British Journal of psychiatry,* 2001; 179: 189-198.

Herpertz S., Werth U., Lukas G., Qunaibi M., Schuerkens A., Kunert H-J., Freese R., Flesch M., Mueller-Isberner R., Osterheider M., Sass H., Emotion in criminal offenders with psychopathy and borderline personality disorder, *Arch. Gen. Psychiatry,* 2001 ; 58: 737-745.

Intrator J., Hare R., Stritzke P., Brichtswein K., Dorfman D., Harpur T., Bernstein D., Handelsman L., Schaefer C., Keilp J., Rosen J., Machac J., A brain imaging (single photon emission computerized tomography) study of semantic and affective processing in psychopaths, *Biol. Psychiatry,* 1997; 42(2): 96-103.

Kaplan and Sadock, Comprehensive book of psychiatry, Seventh edition, Lippincott Williams and Wilkins, 2000.

Kiehl K.A., Smith A.M., Hare R.D., Mendrek A., Forster B.B., Brink J., Liddle P.F., Limbic abnormalities in affective processing by criminal psychopaths as revealed by functional magnetic resonance imaging, *Biol. Psychiatry,* 2001; 50(9): 677-84.

Kim-Cohen J., Caspi A., Moffitt T.E., Harrington H., Milne B.J., Poulton R., Prior juvenile diagnoses in adult with mental disorder: develpmental follow-back of a prospective-longitudinal cohort, *Arch. Gen. Psychiatry,* 2003; 60(7): 709-17.

Kosson DS, Suchy Y, Mayer AR, Libby J, Facial affect recognition in criminal psychopaths, *Emotion,* 2002, 2(4): 398-411.

Laakso M.P., Vaurio O., Koivisto E., Eronen M., Aronen H.J., Hakola P., Repo E., Soininen H., Tiihonen J., Psychopathy and the posterior hippocampus, *Behav. Brain Res,* 2001; 118(2): 187-93.

Lahey B.B., Loeber R., Hart E.L., Frick P.J., Applegate B., Zhang Q., Green S.M., Russo M.F., Four-year longitudinal study of conduct disorder in boys: patterns and predictors of persistence, *J. Abnorm. Psychol,* 1995; 104(1): 83-93.

Lapierre D., Braun C.M., Hodgins S., Ventral frontal deficits in psychopathy: neuropsychological test findings, *Neuropsychologia,* 1995; 33(2): 139-51.

Loeber R., The stability of antisocial and delinquent child behavior: a review., *Child Dev.* 1982 Dec;53(6):1431-46.

Loeber R., Subtypes of conduct disorder., *J. Am. Acad. Child Adolesc. Psychiatry.* 1990 Sep;29(5):837-8.

Loeber R., Antisocial behavior: more enduring than changeable?, *J. Am. Acad. Child Adolesc. Psychiatry.* 1991 May;30(3):393-7.

Loeber R., Burke JD., Lahey BB., What are adolescent antecedents to antisocial personality disorder?, *Crim. Behav. Ment. Health,* 2002; 12(1): 24-36.

Loney BR., Frick PJ., Clements CB., Ellis ML., Kerlin K., Callous-unemotional traits, impulsivity, and emotional processing in adolescents with antisocial behavior problems, *J. Clin. Child Adolesc. Psychol.,* 2003; 32(1): 66-80.

Lynam D.R., Early identification of chronic offenders: who is the fledgling psychopath?, *Psychol. Bull,* 1996; 120(2): 209-34.

Lynam DR, Pursuing the psychopath: Capturing the fledgling psychopath in a nomological net, *J. Abnorm. Psychol,* 1997, 106, 425-438.

Lynam D.R., Early identification of the fledgling psychopath: locating the psychopathic child in the current nomenclature, *J. Abnorm Psychol,* 1998; 107(4): 566-75.

Morgan A.B., Lilienfeld S.O., A meta-analytic review of the relation between antisocial behavior and neuropsychological measures of executive function, *Clin. Psychol. Rev,* 2000; 20(1): 113-36.

Muller JL, Sommer M, Wagner V, Lange K, Taschler H, Roder CH, Schuierer G, Klein HE, Hajak G., Abnormalities in emotion processing within cortical and subcortical regions in criminal psychopaths: evidence from a functional magnetic resonance imaging study using pictures with emotional content., *Biol. Psychiatry.* 2003 Jul 15;54(2):152-62.

Pardini DA, Lochman JE, Frick PJ., Callous/unemotional traits and social-cognitive processes in adjudicated youths, *J. Am. Acad. child. Adolesc. Psychiatry,* 2003, Mar; 42 (3): 364-71.

Patrick C.J., Emotion and psychopathy: startling new insights, *Psychophysiology,* 1994; 31(4): 319-30.

Patrick C.J., Bradley M.M., Lang P.J., Emotion in the criminal psychopath: startle reflex modulation, *J. Aborm. Psychol,* 1993; 102(1): 82-92.

Patrick C.J., Cuthbert B.N., Lang P.J., Emotion in the criminal psychopath: fear image processing, *J. Abnorm. Psychol,* 1994; 103(3): 523-34.

Pelissolo A, Veysseyre O, Lepine JP., Validation of a computerized version of the temperament and character inventory (TCI) in psychiatric inpatients., *Psychiatry Res.* 1997 Oct 10;72(3):195-9.

Pinel, Traité médico-philosophique sur l'aléniation mentale ou la manie, Paris, Richard, Caille and Ravier, an IX, (1801). 2nd edition, Paris, J. A. Brosson, 1809.

Raine A., Biosocial studies of antisocial and violent behavior in children and adults: a review, *J. Abnorm. Child Psychol,* 2002 Aug; 30(4): 311-26.

Raine A, Brennan P, Mednick SA, Bitrh complications with early maternal rejection at age 1 year predispose to violent crime at ge 18 years, *Arch. Gen. Psychiatry,* 1994 Dec; 51(12): 984-8.

Raine A, Brennan P, Mednick B, Mednick SA, High rates of violence, crime, academic problems, and behavioural problems in males with both early neuromotor deficits and unstable family environments, *Arch. Gen. Psychiatry,* 1996 Jun; 53(6): 544-9.

Raine A., Lencz T., Bihrle S., LaCasse L., Colletti P., Reduced prefrontal grey matter volume and reduced autonomic activity in antisocial personality disorder, *Arch. Gen. Psychiatry,* 2000; 57: 119-127.

Raine A, Meloy JR, Bihrle S, Stoddard J, La Casse L, Buchsbaum MS, Reduced prefrontal and increased subcotical brain functioning assessed using positron emission tomography in predatory and affective murderes, *Behav. Sci. Law,* 1998 Summer; 16(3): 319-32.

Raine A, Venables PH, Williams M, High autonomic arousal and electrodermal orienting at age 15 years as protective factors against criminal behavior at age 29 years, *Am. J. Psychiatry,* 1995 Nov; 152 (11): 1595-600.

Raine A, Yaralian PS, Reynolds C, Venables PH, Mednick SA, Spatial but not verbal cognitive deficits at age 3 years in persistently antisocial individuals, *dev. Psychopathol,* 2002 Winter; 14(1): 25-44.

RidgeàPy D, Hare RD., Sensation seeking and psychophysiological responses to auditory stimulation, *Psychophysiology.* 1981 Nov;18(6):613-8.

Schneider K, CLINICAL psychopathology, MW Hamilton, translator, *Grune and Stratton,* New York, 1959.

Schneider F, Habel U, Kessler C, Posse S, Grodd W, Muller-Gartner HW., Functional imaging of conditioned aversive emotional responses in antisocial personality disorder, *Neuropsychobiology.* 2000;42(4):192-201.

Scott S, Knapp M, Henderson J, Maughan B, Financial cost of social exclusion: follow up study of antisocial children into adulthood, *British. Med. Journal,* 2001, 323: 1-5.

Stevens D, Charman T, Blair RJ, Recognition of emotion in facial expressions and vocal tones in children with psychopathic tendencies, *J. Genet Psychol,* 2001, 162(2): 201-11.

Stevens M.C., Kaplan R.F., Hesselbrock V.M., Executive-cognitive functioning in the development of antisocial personality disorder, *Addict Behav,* 2003; 28(2): 285-300.

Stevenson J. and Goodman R., Association between behaviour at age 3 years and adult criminality, *British Journal of psychiatry, 2001*; 179: 197-202.

Thapar A., Harrington R., McGuffin P., Examining the comorbidity of ADHD-related behaviours and conduct problems using a twin study design, *British Journal of psychiatry,* 2001, 179, 224-229.

Veit R., Flor H., Erb M., Hermann C., Lotze M., Grodd W., Birbaumer N., Brain circuits involved in emotional learning in antisocial behavior and social phobia in humans, *Neuroscience Letters,* 328, 2002, 233-236.

Volavka J, Neurobiology of violence. Washington (DC): *American Psychiatric Press,* 1995.

Wakschlag LS, Lahey BB, Loeber R, Green SM, Gordon RA, Leventhal BL, Maternal smoking during pregnancy and the risk of conduct disorder in boys, *Arch. Gen. Psychiatry.* 1997 Jul;54(7):670-6.

Woermann F.G., van Elst L.T., Koepp M.J., Free S.L., Thompson P.J., Trimb M.R., Duncan J.S., Reduction of frontal neocortical grey matter associated with affective aggression in patients with temporal lobe epilepsy: an objective voxel by voxel analysis of automatically segmented MRI, *J. Neurol. Neurosurg. Psychiatry,* 2000; 68(2): 162-9.

Woodworth M, Porter S, In cold blood: characteristics of criminal homicides as a function of psychopathy, *J. Abnorm. Psychol,* 2002; 111(3): 436-45.

INDEX

A

B

D

E

N

O

Q

R

S

T

U

V

W

Y

Z